CONCUSSION

CONCUSSION

A Clinical
Profile Approach
to Assessment
and Treatment

ANTHONY P. KONTOS
MICHAEL W. COLLINS

AMERICAN PSYCHOLOGICAL ASSOCIATION
Washington, DC

Published by
American Psychological Association
750 First Street, NE
Washington, DC 20002
www.apa.org

APA Order Department
P.O. Box 92984
Washington, DC 20090-2984
Phone: (800) 374-2721; Direct: (202) 336-5510
Fax: (202) 336-5502; TDD/TTY: (202) 336-6123
Online: http://www.apa.org/pubs/books
E-mail: order@apa.org

In the U.K., Europe, Africa, and the Middle East, copies may be ordered from
Eurospan Group
c/o Turpin Distribution
Pegasus Drive
Stratton Business Park
Biggleswade Bedfordshire
SG18 8TQ United Kingdom
Phone: +44 (0) 1767 604972
Fax: +44 (0) 1767 601640
Online: https://www.eurospanbookstore.com/apa
E-mail: eurospan@turpin-distribution.com

Typeset in Goudy by Circle Graphics, Inc., Columbia, MD

Printer: Sheridan Books, Chelsea, MI
Cover Designer: Beth Schlenoff Design, Bethesda, MD

Library of Congress Cataloging-in-Publication Data

Names: Kontos, Anthony P., author. | Collins, Michael W. (of University of Pittsburgh. Department of Orthopaedic Surgery), author. | American Psychological Association, issuing body.
Title: Concussion : a clinical profile approach to assessment and treatment / Anthony P. Kontos and Michael W. Collins.
Description: Washington, DC : American Psychological Association, [2018] | Includes bibliographical references and index.
Identifiers: LCCN 2017040908| ISBN 9781433828232 | ISBN 1433828235
Subjects: | MESH: Brain Concussion—diagnosis | Brain Concussion—therapy | Brain Concussion—psychology
Classification: LCC RC394.C7 | NLM WL 354 | DDC 617.4/81044—dc23 LC record available at https://lccn.loc.gov/2017040908

British Library Cataloguing-in-Publication Data
A CIP record is available from the British Library.

Printed in the United States of America
First Edition

http://dx.doi.org/10.1037/0000087-000

10 9 8 7 6 5 4 3 2 1

For my wonderful wife, Danna, and very active children,
Constantine and Marina; for their love and support and for allowing me
to spend Saturday mornings, Friday afternoons, and pretty much all of my
free time writing this book. For my parents, Dino and Doris Kontos,
for their encouragement, love, and support throughout my life and career.
Dad, I finally wrote that book! For my Theo (Uncle) Spyros, for his guidance
and mentoring throughout my life. Thank you to Dr. Valerie Reeves
and Cyndi Holland for their editorial contributions to this book.
—Anthony P. Kontos

Thank you to my wife, Lynn, and our four VERY active girls,
Gabby, Brooke, Payton, and Riley. In the face of a very busy professional
and clinical life, having the love and support of my family is so important.
My family provides the foundational sacrifice, support, and love that
allow me to do my job effectively. I also wish to thank my clinical and
research faculty, fellows and administration at the University of Pittsburgh
Medical Center (UPMC) for providing an environment that is
intellectually curious, fun, supportive, collegial, and so hardworking.
We have an incredible team at UPMC and our collective success is a
by-product of this support, teamwork, and healthy working environment.
Thank you for all the hard work.
—Michael W. Collins

CONTENTS

CONCUSSION

INTRODUCTION

A couple of years ago, the first author of this volume had knee surgery, one of many that was a consequence of a lifetime of playing soccer. This time the surgery involved a microfracture procedure that was a little more involved than previous surgeries and included a long period of physical therapy and rehabilitation. Fortunately, everything went well, and he is now back playing soccer, surfing, hiking, and other physical activities. However, what was interesting about this is the diagnosis that led to the surgery. The diagnosis was a 2-centimeter full-thickness tear in the articular cartilage in the medial compartment of the right knee. As a result of this diagnosis and the subsequent failure of conservative, nonsurgical treatments, an orthopedic surgeon who specializes in knee surgeries recommended the microfracture procedure.

This was a very specific diagnosis of a particular type of knee injury. The orthopedic surgeon did not simply diagnose a "knee injury." Instead, he

http://dx.doi.org/10.1037/0000087-001
Concussion: A Clinical Profile Approach to Assessment and Treatment, by A. P. Kontos and M. W. Collins

diagnosed a subtype ("articular cartilage tear") of knee injury with specific features and characteristics ("2 cm full-thickness . . . medial compartment"). Other diagnoses (e.g., meniscal tear, anterior cruciate ligament tear, dislocation, osteoarthritis, patellar tendon tear) would have resulted in different clinical conceptualization and treatment approaches.

This clinical approach is in stark contrast to the most common approach to diagnosing and conceptualizing a concussion, which is much more homogenous. A homogenous perspective assumes that all concussions are alike and can be treated using a one-size-fits-all approach. But if we have many different types of knee injuries, why would we expect to have one type of concussion? After all, and with no disrespect to knees intended, the brain is infinitely more complex than the knee, yet clinicians and researchers typically rely on a single diagnosis of "concussion."

Unfortunately, current conceptual approaches to assessing and treating concussion continue to revolve around this faulty homogenous perspective. This homogenous perspective is, in part, to blame for the numerous failed clinical trials for treating concussion (Z. Zhang, Larner, Kobeissy, Hayes, & Wang, 2010). In each of these trials, the researchers have conceptualized concussion from a homogenous perspective involving symptoms and perhaps cognitive or balance impairment. The key assumption in these studies is that a specific pharmacological therapy will improve symptoms and impairment of *all* patients with a concussion in the same manner. However, as evident in the failure of these trials, the reality is that these therapies are likely improving symptoms and impairment in a small subsample of patients. This subsample might have in common specific symptoms, impairment, risk factors, or other characteristics, thereby resulting in a successful outcome following therapy. In contrast, patients with different symptoms, impairment, and other characteristics may experience no benefit or an adverse response to the same therapy, and thus, the trials fail.

Similarly, in the growing literature in concussion, the majority of empirical studies include one or more of the following outcome variables: total symptoms or symptom severity, cognitive, or balance impairment. As a result of this generalized approach (from which all concussions are measured the same way) the effect sizes or magnitude of changes reported that are related to the effects of concussion are often minimized. Again, the issue is that not all patients have the same symptoms and impairments. It was not until recently that researchers began to expand the outcomes assessed following concussion to include vestibular (e.g., Mucha et al., 2014), oculomotor (e.g., Pearce, Sufrinko, et al., 2015), psychological (e.g., Kontos, Covassin, Elbin, & Parker, 2012), and other outcomes. However, the majority of researchers continue to select the same outcomes in their studies, leading to less robust findings and potentially missing the true effects associated with this injury.

Although concussions may share some underlying biomechanical and pathophysiological characteristics, even these similar underpinnings may lead to different outcomes. These different outcomes may result from a variety of risk factors, and these differences cannot be boiled down to a total symptom score or only balance impairment. We typically measure more than 20 different symptoms associated with this injury that range from dizziness, headache, and nausea to trouble concentrating and sleep problems. Symptom presentation alone provides compelling evidence that concussion is a highly individualized injury that demands a conceptual framework that goes beyond the current one-size-fits-all approach.

DEFINING CONCUSSION

In developing our own definition of concussion, we began by considering a typical definition representative of the field: "a traumatic brain injury induced by biomechanical forces" (P. McCrory et al., 2017, p. 2). The definition goes on to describe concussion as involving direct and impulsive (i.e., indirect) forces to the head, short-lived impairment, evolving initial signs and symptoms, functional versus structural injury, and a range of clinical signs and symptoms. Although the initial portion of this definition is succinct and provides a conceptual framework for this injury, it lacks operational or practical application and does not reflect our evolving understanding of this injury. We thus propose to extend the above definition as follows:

> a complex pathophysiological process affecting the brain, induced by biomechanical forces, *which may involve different symptoms, impairment, clinical profiles or subtypes, and recovery trajectories that are influenced by a variety of risk factors.*

We believe that this definition of concussion represents a more accurate and practical reflection of the current thinking regarding this injury. We address concussion terminology in more detail in Chapter 2.

GOALS AND ROADMAP OF THIS BOOK

The primary objective of this book is to present and discuss an evidence-based, targeted, and comprehensive approach to concussion assessment and care that accounts for the heterogeneous nature of the injury. This approach incorporates a comprehensive assessment, an interdisciplinary approach, and targeted, active treatments. It is based on our 30 plus years of collective experience in concussion clinical care and research.

Because the approach relies on a health care team with diverse specialties, this book is intended for any professional who might be involved in concussion care, including athletic trainers, clinical/counseling psychologists, neuropsychologists, neurologists, neurosurgeons, optometrists, physical therapists, and primary care physicians. We realize that in many instances, it is not feasible or possible (for reasons of geography, access to health care, or financial constraints) to assemble a comprehensive team of interdisciplinary health professionals. In fact, it is more common that a single health care provider is responsible for all aspects of concussions clinical care rather than an integrated, interdisciplinary team. However, through the cultivation of proper referral networks and the growing field of telemedicine, these barriers can be overcome. Regardless of whether a patient is treated by a team or an individual, the information in this book provides a guide to better understand, conceptualize, and treat this injury from an interdisciplinary perspective.

We hope that this book acts as a catalyst to advance the discussion about concussion such that more comprehensive, active, and targeted approaches to assessing and treating concussion become the standard of care moving forward. In short, we believe concussion is a treatable injury and that when it is managed properly and in a timely fashion, a positive outcome can result.

We have organized this book in a progressive manner with a focus on understanding this injury. The first few chapters help conceptualize concussion. We begin with an overview of our model, emphasizing the six clinical profiles (Chapter 1). We then provide a broader review of how concussion functions, including underlying mechanics and pathophysiology, as well as common signs and symptoms. We refer to this review as "Concussion 101," and it reinforces the approach we propose in this book (Chapter 2). We then review the psychological issues related to concussion (Chapter 3). Next, we apply this understanding to clinical practice. We provide a comprehensive approach to assessment (Chapter 4) and targeted, active treatment and rehabilitation strategies (Chapter 5). We also present and discuss case examples that represent the various clinical profiles to better illustrate the model in action (Chapter 6). Finally, we examine more closely specific at-risk groups and issues related to concussion (Chapter 7) and consider where the field is heading (Chapter 8).

1

OVERVIEW OF THE MODEL

This chapter presents an overview of our model for the treatment of concussion, including the six clinical profiles, the interdisciplinary team, and the focus on targeted active treatment. To provide context, we begin with a brief review of the traditional homogenous approach to concussion.

HOMOGENOUS APPROACH TO CONCUSSION

Traditionally, concussion has been conceptualized and managed from a homogenous perspective that has permeated the concussion research literature and has been the driving framework for clinical approaches to managing concussion. As a result, initial attempts to characterize and treat concussion focused on grading scales that were predicated on the presence of specific signs and symptoms of the injury, including amnesia, disorientation/confusion,

http://dx.doi.org/10.1037/0000087-002
Concussion: A Clinical Profile Approach to Assessment and Treatment, by A. P. Kontos and M. W. Collins
Copyright © 2018 by the American Psychological Association. All rights reserved.

balance problems, and, in particular, loss of consciousness (LOC; Cantu, 1986, 2001; Kelly & Rosenberg, 1997).

However, we now know that fewer than 10% of concussions involve LOC (Guskiewicz, Weaver, Padua, & Garrett, 2000). Moreover, brief (< 1 minute) LOC has not been shown to be a consistent predictor of outcome severity or duration (Lovell, Iverson, Collins, McKeag, & Maroon, 1999; P. McCrory et al., 2013). In fact, in a study of time of injury predictors or recovery time following concussion, we reported that LOC and vomiting were protective factors for concussion recovery time (i.e., patients who had brief LOC or vomited recovered faster than those who had neither characteristic; Lau, Kontos, Collins, Mucha, & Lovell, 2011). At first glance, this finding may seem to be counterintuitive. However, two explanations for this seemingly anomalous finding can be proposed:

1. These overt signs of the injury result in more conservative decision making and management by medical professionals.
2. Brief LOC may insulate the brain from the metabolic effects of this injury by reducing energy demands during the critical first few moments of a concussion. Longer duration LOC (e.g., 5 minutes) is an important predictor of a more severe brain injury (i.e., moderate traumatic brain injury [TBI]) and poorer outcomes (Jennett & Bond, 1975).

Another consequence of a homogenous approach to concussion has been the assumption that because all concussions are similar, they can be treated with one management strategy. The most prominent strategy for concussion is prescribed physical and cognitive rest. However, this approach to treatment for patients with a concussion is based largely on expert consensus (Giza et al., 2013; P. McCrory et al., 2013), with limited empirical evidence to support it. In fact, the 2013 Institute of Medicine and National Research Council report on concussion in sport states, "there is little evidence regarding the efficacy of rest following concussion or to inform the best timing and approach for return to activity" and recommends "randomized controlled trials (RCT) . . . to determine the efficacy of physical or cognitive rest" (Institute of Medicine & National Research Council, 2014, p. 13).

Rest is an intuitive and widely embraced therapy for many medical conditions. The theory for rest suggests that during a period of increased metabolic demand and limited adenosine triphosphate (ATP) reserves (as occurs after concussion), cognitive and physical activity may require oxygen and ATP from recovering neurons. However, a review of research on rest, long considered "intuitive" for recovery from many medical conditions, showed rest to be ineffective in all conditions studied (Allen, Glasziou, & Del Mar, 1999). One of only two published randomized clinical trials of rest for treatment of concussion, comparing no rest versus 6 days of bed rest in 107 adults, showed no benefit to rest (de Kruijk, Leffers, Meerhoff, Rutten, & Twijnstra, 2002). Patients with chronic concussive symptoms may in fact benefit from more active rehabilitation (e.g., low-level physical activity; P. McCrory et al., 2013). Our colleagues at the Medical College of Wisconsin recently completed a study of 99 pediatric patients in the emergency department in which they found that cognitive and physical rest for 5 days following concussion did not improve neurocognitive or symptom outcomes (D. G. Thomas, Apps, Hoffmann, McCrea, & Hammeke, 2015). In fact, some patients in this study benefitted more from more active strategies, whereas others benefitted from rest. These findings add further support to the notion that concussion is not a homogenous injury; it should be viewed as a heterogeneous disorder that requires an individualized clinical approach.

AN ANALOGY BETWEEN CONCUSSIONS AND WAVES

Many concussion researchers and clinicians compare the individual nature of concussions to that of snowflakes, with no two being alike. However, we think an analogy to breaking waves may be more fitting. Despite their seemingly similar appearance on the surface, no two ocean waves are alike, again much like concussions. Breaking waves can be of different height, thickness, direction, and speed depending on a variety of factors from the wind and fetch (i.e., the distance the wind has to blow and act on the waves) to what lies beneath the surface and the shape of the coastline. Nevertheless, sets and patterns of breaking waves that share similar characteristics are evident and can be grouped together into similar types, such as point break, beach break, and submerged reef.

Regardless of the shared characteristics, each breaking wave is uniquely shaped by the environment—the nature of the wave and coastline, including characteristics that are readily visible on the surface, in addition to those that are under the surface—ocean floor contours, reefs, sand bars, and rocks. Similarly, concussions are shaped by known (e.g., age, sex, concussion history) and unknown (e.g., genetics, undiagnosed migraine or motion sickness) risk factors (see Figure 1.1). Moreover, much like a "set wave" (i.e., one that is much larger and faster than other breaking waves in a set) can come out of nowhere and have devastating consequences, so too can a seemingly straightforward impact to the head result in a substantial concussion with a prolonged and complicated recovery. However, just like a set wave has certain factors that combine to increase its likelihood and effects, so too do patients have certain risk factors that increase their likelihood that one concussion will have substantial adverse effects. Just as certain types of waves share characteristics,

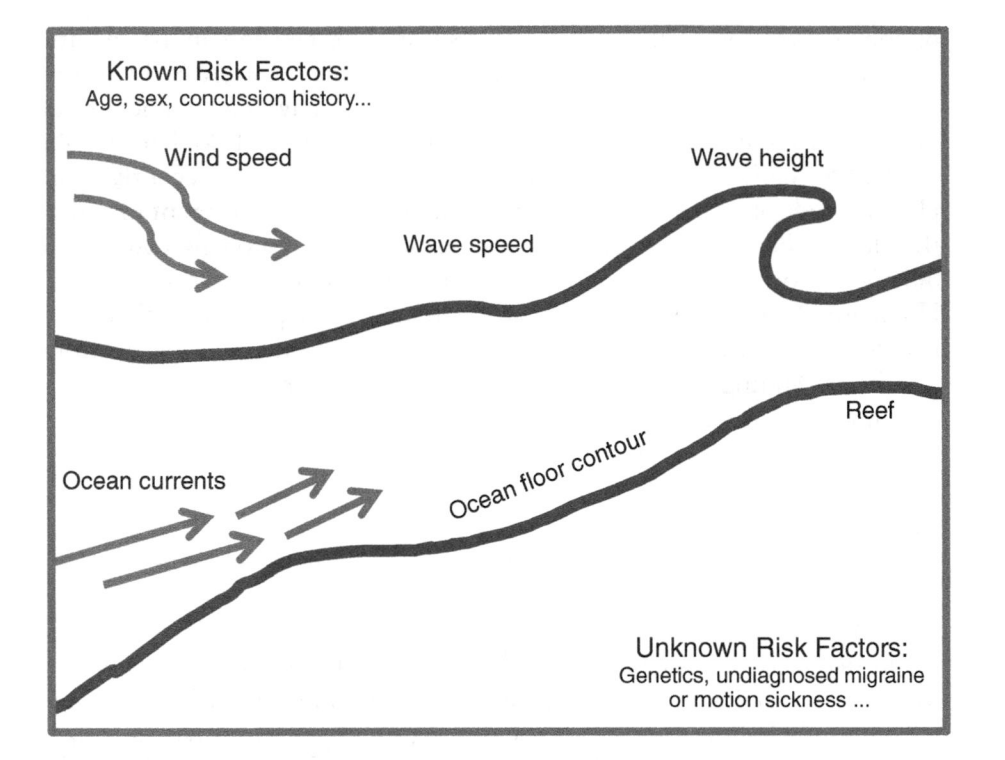

Figure 1.1. Wave analogy for concussions.

so too do certain types of concussions. Therefore, to provide a systematic approach to this heterogeneous injury, we focus on the shared characteristics of clinical profiles of concussions. However, in so doing, we are mindful that certain risk or modifying factors may mitigate or exacerbate these characteristics in each patient (see Chapter 2).

HETEROGENEITY: BUILDING A CASE FOR CLINICAL PROFILES

Because a majority of patients with concussion recover spontaneously within 2 to 3 weeks after an injury, people often erroneously assume that most concussions are similar and do not require any specific treatment. As a result, approaches to care during the early postinjury phases primarily consist of rest-based interventions. Specifically, it is recommended in concussion consensus documents that patients rest both physically and cognitively during the initial postinjury period with a gradual return to activity based on symptoms (e.g., P. McCrory et al., 2013, 2017). Some of these consensus documents expand this notion to include symptom specific management strategies as needed (e.g., National Collegiate Athletic Association Sport Science Institute, 2016), but that is the extent of treatment.

This approach is somewhat surprising given that symptom factors or clusters have been used to describe patients' experiences following concussion since the early 2000s (e.g., Pardini et al., 2004; see also Chapter 2, this volume). These earlier attempts at categorizing concussion were based on symptoms only and described three or four symptom factors: cognitive, somatic (or physical), affective (or emotional), and sleep-related (e.g., Pardini et al., 2004). In a more recent study in which we focused on symptoms only in the first week after the injury, we uncovered a more global symptom factor early on in the injury process (Kontos, Elbin, et al., 2012), suggesting that concussion symptoms may evolve into more distinct factors later on in the injury process. As a result of the complex and individual symptom presentation following concussion, together with previous and in many cases ineffective one-size-fits-all approaches to managing concussion, researchers and clinicians alike have responded with a more heterogeneous framework to understand and subsequently treat this injury.

A NEW APPROACH TO UNDERSTANDING CONCUSSION

Clinical Profiles

In 2014, we proposed a new conceptual approach to understanding concussion that involves six clinical profiles (previously referred to as *clinical trajectories* or *clinical subtypes*). A concussion clinical profile, which may be referred to as a clinical subtype, clinical trajectory or phenotype, is characterized in patients by a similar set of symptoms, impairment, risk factors, and other characteristics and clinical outcomes. The six clinical profiles are vestibular, oculomotor, cognitive/fatigue, PTM, anxiety/mood, and cervical (M. W. Collins, Kontos, Reynolds, Murawski, & Fu, 2014; see Figure 1.2). An additional component of the clinical profiles is sleep disruption, which may also affect patients with concussion but does not appear to be a distinct profile onto itself. Consequently, sleep deficits are likely to affect some patients following a concussion and may warrant assessment from clinicians (P. McCrory et al., 2013). However, this component is not considered a separate profile, but rather a modifier that may occur concurrently with and affect the other profiles. In short, patients with this injury may experience sleep disruption regardless of the specific concussion clinical profiles they may have.

Clinical profiles are less distinct within the first week of the injury process because concussion presents as a more "global" phenomenon characterized

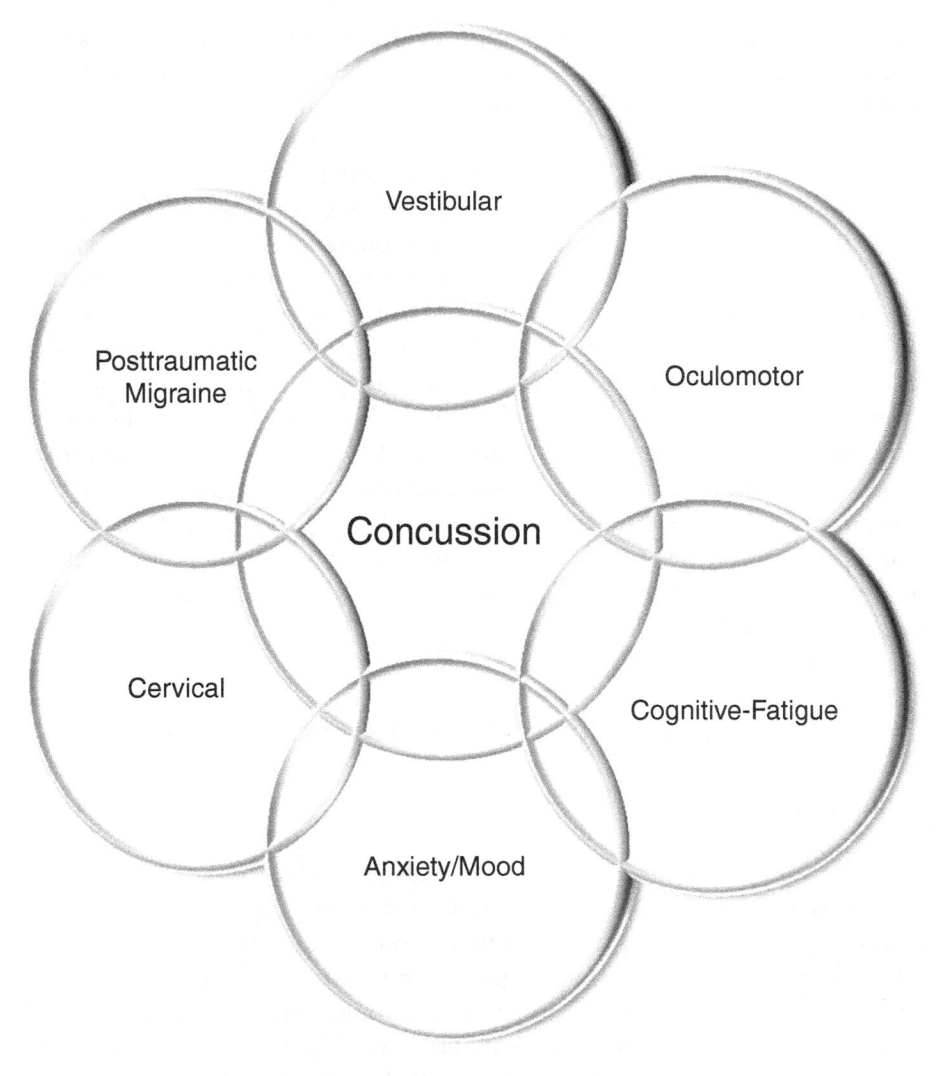

Figure 1.2. Clinical profiles for concussion. From "A Comprehensive, Targeted Approach to the Clinical Care of Athletes Following Sport-Related Concussion," by M. W. Collins, A. P. Kontos, E. Reynolds, C. D. Murawski, and F. H. Fu, 2014, *Knee Surgery, Sports Traumatology, Arthroscopy, 22*, p. 240. Copyright 2014 by Springer. Adapted with permission.

by a primary cognitive-fatigue-migraine cluster of symptoms during this time (Kontos, Elbin, et al., 2012). Nonetheless, in our experience a comprehensive assessment can help to uncover evidence for potential pathways in patients even during the first week of injury. It is important to conduct a comprehensive assessment and follow-up with patients within a week of their initial presentation to confirm initial clinical impressions to drive targeted treatments.

Each clinical profile is not mutually exclusive and may share some symptoms and impairments with other profiles. As a result of this overlap in symptoms and impairment together with the somewhat global presentation of symptoms during the first week after the injury (discussed in Chapter 2), clinical profiles become more distinct following the first week of injury. Consequently, it is ideal to evaluate patients both during the first few days following the injury, as well as 1 to 2 weeks following injury when clinical profiles typically become more clearly defined.

The clinical profiles approach integrates the authors' more than 15 years of clinical experience treating concussion with growing evidence that concussions have distinct clinical profiles, many of which may be amenable to targeted and early treatments. However, it is important to note that our understanding and conceptualization of each clinical profile continue to evolve. In fact, many of our clinical profiles did not yet exist even a few years ago or were demonstrably different from those we use today. As empirical evidence continues to grow and change, our concussion clinical profiles will also continue to evolve. We are currently working with researchers and clinicians to revise the clinical profiles and develop an evidence-based approach to quantifying them for clinical and research purposes. Regardless, we think it is important to describe briefly the clinical profiles in their current form to better understand this new approach to conceptualizing and treating this injury and the premise for the rest of the book. We have also included information about the clinical profiles and concurrent risk factors that are often associated with each profile

Vestibular

The vestibular clinical profile involves the disruption of the central vestibular system and is characterized by symptoms such as dizziness, vertigo, fogginess, detachment, and nausea. Impairments in the vestibular clinical profile include visual motion sensitivity or problems with maintaining gaze stability while moving the head up and down or side to side; balance problems (though these are often absent), and slowed reaction time and processing speed.

Risk factors for the vestibular clinical profile include a history of motion sickness or other vestibular disorders, migraine headaches, and dizziness at the time of injury. Individuals with the vestibular profile may often have one or more of the following concurrent clinical profiles: posttraumatic migraine, anxiety/mood, and oculomotor.

Oculomotor

The oculomotor clinical profile involves disruption of the brain's coordination of the visual system and input, and may include symptoms such as blurry or double vision, attentional problems, fatigue, and headaches (especially when reading). Impairments may include convergence or accommodative insufficiency, inability to perform smooth pursuits or saccadic eye movements, difficulty reading, vision dependent academic/work deficits, slowed reaction time, and decrements in visual memory. The patient with an oculomotor clinical profile may be initially misdiagnosed as having a cognitive clinical profile based on the impairments. Therefore, it is important to consider the visual system whenever cognitive deficits are evident.

Risk factors for the oculomotor clinical profile include a history of vision problems. Individuals with the oculomotor profile often also have a cognitive-fatigue or posttraumatic migraine (or both) clinical profile.

Cognitive-Fatigue

The cognitive-fatigue clinical profile involves a general worsening of symptoms throughout the day and may include symptoms such as headache (that worsens with cognitive activity and throughout the day), lack of energy, fatigue or drowsiness, and sleep disruption. Impairments may include general decreases in performance on neurocognitive tasks, concentration and attentional focus that worsen throughout the day, and academic or work performance that is worse as the day goes on.

Risk factors for the cognitive-fatigue clinical profile include learning disability, attention-deficit/hyperactivity disorder. Individuals with the cognitive-fatigue profile might not have a concurrent clinical profile.

Posttraumatic Migraine

The hallmark symptoms of the posttraumatic migraine (PTM) profile include headache, nausea, and photosensitivity and/or phonosensitivity. Other symptoms may include stress, changes in mood, decreased activity levels, and sleep disruption. Impairments may include memory deficits, particularly on visual memory tasks. In cases where PTM is related to vestibular or ocular provocation, these impairments and symptoms may exist.

Risk factors for the PTM clinical profile include a history of motion sickness or other vestibular disorders or migraine headaches. Individuals with the PTM profile may often have one or more of the following concurrent clinical profiles: vestibular, oculomotor, or anxiety/mood.

Anxiety/Mood

The anxiety/mood clinical profile involves changes in mood, including feelings of nervousness/anxiety and/or sadness/depression along with the concomitant hallmark symptoms of these mood disturbances. For nervousness/anxiety, these symptoms may include racing or intrusive thoughts, hypervigilance, worry, edginess, and sleep disruption. For sadness/depression, these symptoms may include feelings of hopelessness, irritability/anger, overwhelmed, loss of energy, fatigue, and sleep disruption. Impairments are generally absent, but some patients may experience provoked symptoms with vestibular and oculomotor testing.

Risk factors for the anxiety/mood clinical profile include history of mood disorder. Individuals with the anxiety/mood profile often have a vestibular or PTM (or both) clinical profile.

Cervical

Patients with a cervical clinical profile have an underlying cervicogenic component to their concussion as a result of the neck's involvement during the injury process or preexisting cervical vulnerability. These patients may present with a variety of symptoms, including headache, neck pain, and numbness/tingling. Headaches for this profile often emanate from the back of the head. Impairments are often absent for patients with this profile.

Risk factors for the cervical clinical profile include an injury involving the neck or a preexisting cervical vulnerability. Individuals with the cervical profile might have a concurrent anxiety/mood clinical profile.

Note About Sleep

Although sleep disruption may occur with some clinical profiles (e.g., anxiety/mood, cervical, PTM), we do not believe that sleep disruption constitutes a separate clinical profile, nor is it ubiquitous with concussion. In fact, only 33% of patients experience sleep disruption (Kontos, Elbin, et al., 2012). We believe that sleep disruption is a common symptom that may co-occur with other clinical profiles. Sleep disruptions may involve sleep frequency (insomnia or hypersomnia) or sleep quality (sleep initiation, completion of sleep cycles, parasomnia). Sleep disruptions may be acute and resolve as symptoms improve, or they may become chronic and persist even as symptoms abate. In any case, any sleep disruption should be treated immediately; if it persists it may prolong recovery and limit the effectiveness of other therapies.

Prioritizing Clinical Profiles

Although some patients may present with a single clinical profile such as oculomotor or vestibular only, others may present with two or more clinical profiles simultaneously. For example, a patient may have vestibular and PTM clinical profiles; or vestibular and anxiety/mood; or PTM and anxiety/mood; or oculomotor and cognitive-fatigue; or vestibular and oculomotor and PTM. Therefore, it is important to not only assess and identify the various concussion clinical profiles but also to prioritize which clinical profile is most pronounced and requires more immediate treatment. To do this, we conceptualize profiles as being primary, secondary, or tertiary (see Figure 1.3). This hierarchy informs treatment timing and allows for more targeted approaches to expedite a patient's recovery.

Primary profiles involve the most pronounced and obvious clinical characteristics or represent the profile that underlies secondary and tertiary issues. As such, the primary profile should be treated first. Treatment of secondary and tertiary profiles, while important to ensure good clinical outcomes, is secondary to treatment of the primary profile. Prioritization of clinical profiles into primary, secondary, and tertiary flows from the information gathered during the clinical interview, comprehensive assessments, time since injury, and other factors. The interrelationships among symptoms and impairment may also drive prioritization. For instance, a patient with PTM may experience migraine-like headaches that provoke anxiety. In this case, treating the PTM would take priority over the anxiety/mood treatment. Similarly, a patient may have vestibular symptoms such as dizziness or vertigo that result in anxiety from the uncontrollable nature of the onset of the vestibular symptoms.

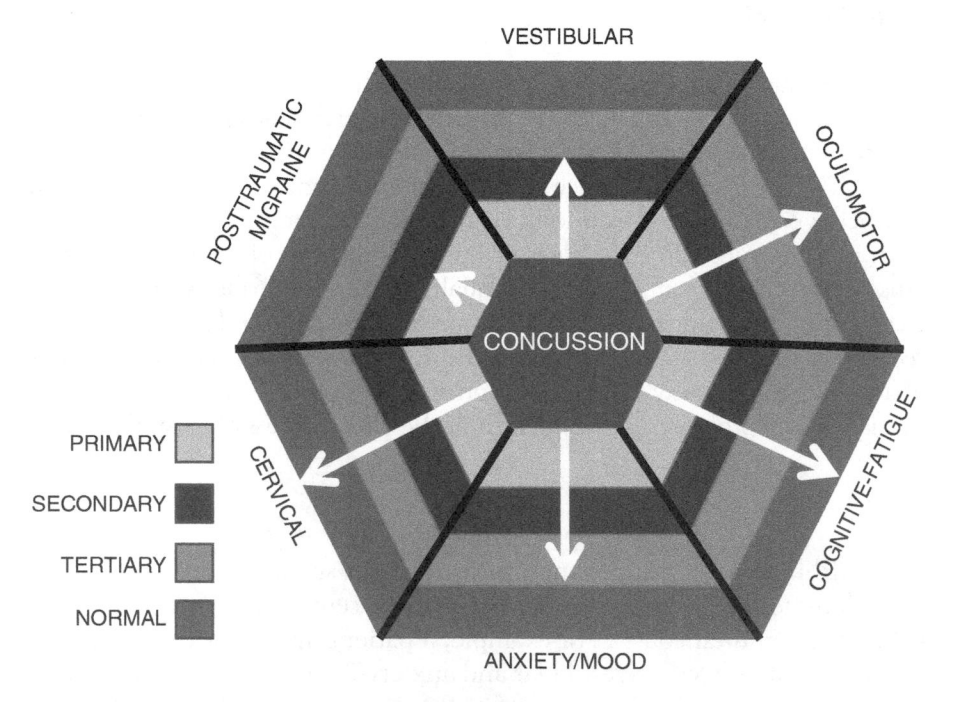

Figure 1.3. Example of primary, secondary, and tertiary clinical profiles to help prioritize treatment and rehabilitation strategies.

Again, in this case, the underlying vestibular impairment and symptoms would be treated first. In addition, preexisting risk factors, such as a history of migraine or motion sickness, may influence which trajectory needs to be treated first. It is also important to point out that sleep disruption, which may accompany several different clinical profiles, may need to be treated concurrently with the primary trajectory. If sleep disruptions are ignored or not treated, the effectiveness of interventions for the primary profile may be negated.

PUTTING IT ALL TOGETHER: A COMPREHENSIVE CLINICAL PROFILE-BASED MODEL FOR CONCUSSION

Earlier we intimated that concussions are like breaking waves; no two are the same, but they can be categorized and to some extent predicted on the basis of a variety of characteristics such as the shape of the ocean floor, underwater structures, wind direction and speed, and direction of the swell. However, each wave remains unique, and as a result cannot be totally "figured out" using information from similar previous waves, even in the exact same spot, as any surfer will readily confirm. So, while we can identify similarities across patients with similar concussion clinical profiles, we cannot adopt a cookie cutter approach to understanding and treating this heterogeneous injury.

Previously, we described a comprehensive clinical profile model for understanding concussion that emphasized the role of risk factors, the injury, and subsequent clinical profiles in determining appropriate targeted treatment pathways (see M. W. Collins, Kontos, Reynolds, Murawski, & Fu, 2014; M. W. Collins et al., 2016). We believe that this evolving model allows for an individualized, patient-centered approach for treatment of this injury that takes into account the variability in this injury. Such an approach, although systematic, does not represent a cookie cutter approach and respects the individualized nature of each concussion and patient. If we go back to the wave analogy, to better understand a wave's characteristics, one must adopt a comprehensive approach to assess meteorologic, oceanographic, geographic, hydrologic, and other components that make up the wave. Similarly, to understand a concussion's characteristics requires a comprehensive assessment of neurological, psychological, cervical, vestibular, ocular, and other components. Therefore, several components are key to the successful implementation of the current model for assessing and treating patients with concussion: a comprehensive assessment; an interdisciplinary approach; and targeted, active treatments. A brief overview of the importance of each of these topics follows.

Comprehensive Assessment

To appropriately determine a patient's clinical profile or profiles, one must have a comprehensive approach to the assessment of a concussion combining the breadth of information from formal assessment tools that cover multiple domains of concussion outcomes (e.g., symptoms, cognitive, vestibular, oculomotor) with the depth of information from clinical interviews (M. W. Collins et al., 2014). A concurrent assessment of preexisting risk factors (e.g., concussion, history, migraine, motion sickness) should also accompany the assessment of the injury and its effects to provide insight into potential clinical pathways of the injury. The purpose of such an approach is to identify, conceptualize, and prioritize for treatment a patient's clinical profiles following concussion. The comprehensive assessment should help screen for additional, more in-depth profiles-specific assessments. For example, positive screening for psychological, vestibular, and vision deficits would be followed with referrals to a licensed health care provider with expertise in the area of the particular deficit. The comprehensive assessment, including the clinical interview, symptoms, neurocognitive, vestibular, oculomotor, and neuroimaging and emerging components, is discussed in depth in Chapter 4.

Interdisciplinary Approach

Given that concussions are highly individualized and involve numerous symptoms and functional impairments, an interdisciplinary approach to this injury is warranted. In short, ideally the most interdisciplinary approach would involve a team of experts from various disciplines to properly assess and treat this injury. This team would comprise health professionals from the following complementary disciplines: athletic training, clinical/counseling psychology, neuropsychology, neurology, neurosurgery, optometry, physical therapy, and primary care physicians (see Figure 1.4). In addition to their own areas of expertise, these individuals should each have specialized training in concussion care. Developing a network of local and national referrals is critical to the success of any concussion team. However, one does not need a large team of experts to employ an interdisciplinary approach to concussion. We realize that in many instances, it is not feasible or possible (because of geography, access to health care, or financial constraints) to assemble a comprehensive team of interdisciplinary health professionals. In fact, it is more common that a single health care provider is responsible for all aspects of concussion clinical care rather than an integrated, interdisciplinary team. However, through the cultivation of proper referral networks and the growing field of telemedicine, these barriers can be overcome moving forward. Regardless of whether a patient is treated by a team or an individual, the information in this book

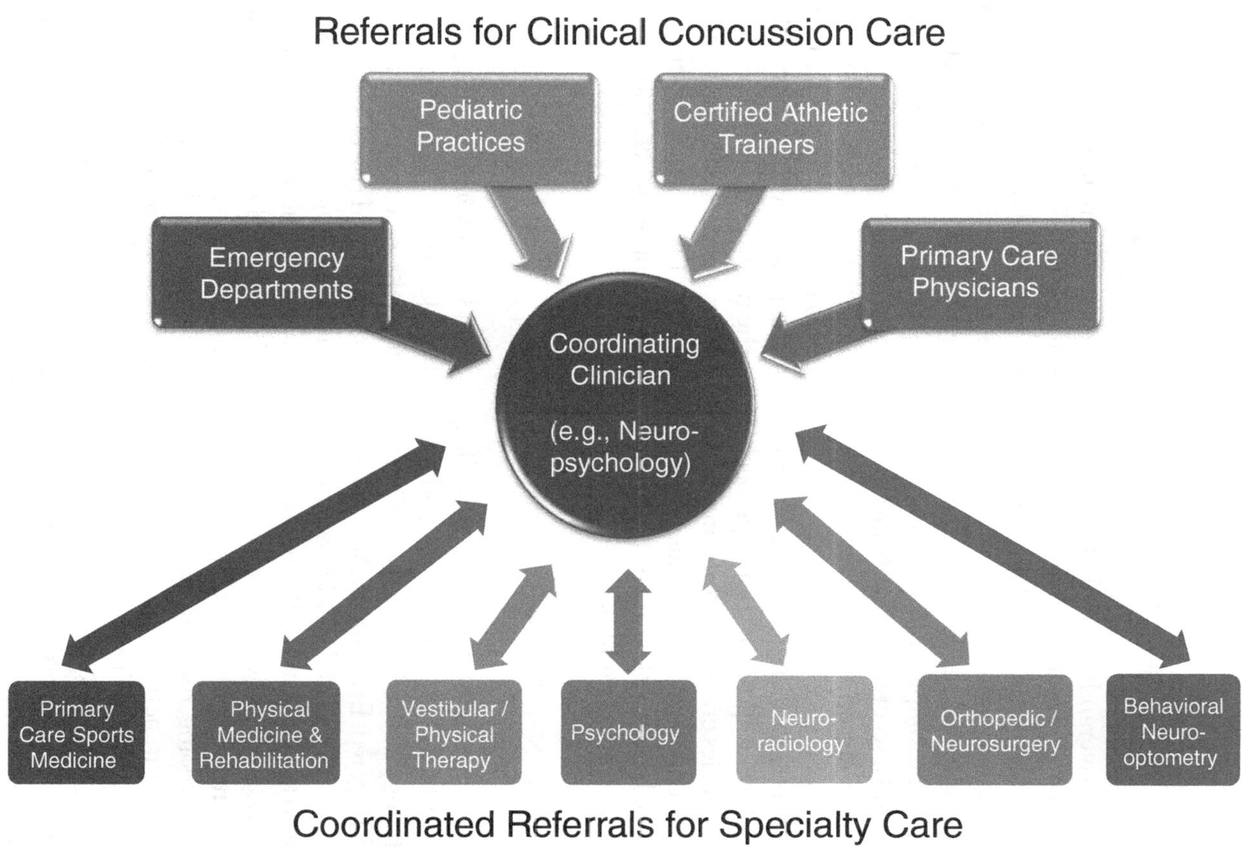

Referrals for Clinical Concussion Care

Figure 1.4. The interdisciplinary concussion team.

Coordinated Referrals for Specialty Care

provides a guide to better understand, conceptualize, and treat this injury from an interdisciplinary perspective. The roles of different health care providers (including psychologists) for clinical concussion care are discussed in more detail in Chapter 5.

Targeted Treatment Pathways

The overarching goal of a comprehensive assessment and determination of clinical profiles for concussion is to inform targeted treatment pathways to reduce impairment and symptoms and recovery time. Effective management of concussion, we believe, requires matching up active treatment and rehabilitation strategies to the patient's clinical profiles (M. W. Collins et al., 2014). For example, a concussion patient with a primary vestibular clinical profile and a secondary anxiety profile might receive specific active treatments and rehabilitation strategies, including dynamic exertion therapies and vestibular exercises, in addition to behavioral strategies to reduce anxiety. Note that the treatments would be prioritized to address the primary vestibular profile first. A key component of this approach is that the treatments and rehabilitation strategies are active compared with the passive prescribed rest approach typically employed with concussions (Broglio et al., 2015). Chapter 5 includes additional information about targeted, active treatment approaches for each of the six clinical profiles.

Testing the New Model

In 2014, we—along with our colleagues David Okonkwo in the Department of Neurological Surgery and Walt Schneider in the Department of Psychology at the University of Pittsburgh—started a new research project titled Targeted, Evaluation, Action and Monitoring (TEAM) of TBI that was funded through the U.S. Department of Defense. The objective of TEAM TBI is to use clinical profiles to conceptualize and inform subsequent targeted treatments for patients with chronic mild TBI. We are also measuring the effectiveness of targeted treatments to determine which ones are most effective. In so doing, the study has afforded us an opportunity to characterize clinical profiles in active duty and retired military personnel, as well as civilian patients with mild TBI.

One unique aspect of TEAM TBI is its focus on conducting not only clinical and behavioral assessments of patients but also cutting-edge neuroimaging, including MRI, high-definition fiber tracking (HDFT), magnetoencephalography (MEG), and positron emission tomography (PET) scans. Therefore, the study is allowing us to see whether neuroimaging findings correspond to clinical and behavioral findings and support the clinical profiles. Similarly, we recently concluded a study (W. Schneider et al., 2014) with the same colleagues from TEAM TBI that used high-definition fiber tracking (which identifies brain tracts associated with specific functions) to corroborate clinical profile findings in young athletes with sport-related concussions. This study, which was funded through the Head Health Initiative jointly supported by General Electric (GE) and the National Football League (NFL), has provided initial support for correlations between clinical impairment and damage to white matter in specific brain tracts. Both the TEAM TBI and GE-NFL Head Health Initiative projects represent good first steps in providing empirical support for the clinical profile models described here. However, additional research is needed to better characterize and quantify the current and evolving clinical profiles moving forward.

ALTERNATE APPROACHES

Although our conceptual approach using the six clinical profiles was the first such approach to be published and has gained support among clinicians and researchers, other researchers have proposed clinical profile-based conceptual approaches to this injury (Ellis, Leddy, & Willer, 2015). In their conceptual model, Ellis, Leddy, and Willer (2015) proposed three distinct concussion disorders, as they call them: physiological, vestibulo-ocular, and cervicogenic. These researchers also included two postconcussion modifying factors: posttraumatic mood and PTM. These concussion disorders and modifying factors share some similarities in both name and characteristics with some of our six clinical profiles; however, the two approaches have several key differences. Most important, this approach relies on exercise-induced symptom reporting and physical response in addition to patient's medical history to determine clinical profiles. In addition, patients cannot be determined to have a disorder or modifying factor until 3 weeks after an injury. As such, early intervention for patients is minimized, thereby potentially and unnecessarily prolonging their recovery. Finally, the approach of Ellis and colleagues does not address potential overlap or prioritization of disorders or modifying factors. Despite these shortcomings, this model offers an alternative, profile-based conceptual approach to working with patients with concussion that goes beyond the current one-size-fits-all approaches.

Researchers who specialize in cervical spinal injuries have speculated that much of what is reported to be concussion is actually cervical in nature (Leslie & Craton, 2013). These researchers reference the clinical manifestation and literature on whiplash-associated disorder (WAD) as support for their claim. They believe that symptoms of concussion are indiscernible from symptoms of WAD, and as such, many concussions are actually WAD. Again, although these researchers make a valid point that many concussions involve the cervical spine, they do not provide evidence that most concussions are in fact cervical in origin. However, these researchers do accurately point out that misdiagnosing a noncervical concussion and prescribing rest—instead of more active physical therapy-based rehabilitations strategies—may be counterproductive and prolong the recovery process. Although we do not believe that most concussions are cervical in nature, we do agree that it is important to assess the cervical spine following any suspected concussion and that the cervical cluster of symptoms represents a separate clinical profile for patients with this injury.

CONCLUSION

The field of concussion has experienced tremendous and accelerated growth during the past decade. Surprisingly, and despite this increase in knowledge about concussion, the way in which concussions are conceptualized and treated continues to be mired in the past. Much of the research on concussion and the clinical approach to treating this injury is based on a dated homogenous approach wherein treatments and management strategies are applied with limited regard to the different presentations for patients with this injury. This one-size-fits-all approach is reflective of, or more accurately derived from, the static nature of the current consensus and standard of care statements, which fail to address the heterogeneity and complex, individual nature of this injury. Until the discussion and approach to conceptualizing and treating concussion is moved forward in a more progressive manner based on the characteristics of the injury, patient risk factors, and comprehensive assessment outcomes, treatment and management of this injury will continue to evolve at a snail's pace. In the meantime, many patients with concussion will continue to receive ineffective care that results in unnecessarily poor and prolonged adverse outcomes.

2

CONCUSSION 101

This chapter provides readers with a broad understanding of key concussion concepts that lay the foundation for understanding this injury and the information discussed in subsequent chapters. We present historical and modern views on concussion, including ways that this injury magnifies preexisting conditions. Along the way, we explore the underlying mechanics, pathophysiology, signs, and symptoms. We highlight the role of established and emerging risk factors to provide context for the development of different clinical profiles and outcomes associated with concussion.

WHY CONCUSSION?

Not too long ago (think late 1990s or early 2000s), concussions—particularly when they occurred in the context of sport—were viewed by medical professionals, athletes, and others as a nuisance injury or not an

http://dx.doi.org/10.1037/0000087-003
Concussion: A Clinical Profile Approach to Assessment and Treatment, by A. P. Kontos and M. W. Collins
Copyright © 2018 by the American Psychological Association. All rights reserved.

injury at all. In fact, concussions were perceived as no more severe or conse-quential than a bruise or twisted ankle and were often referred to as a "bell ringer," "ding," or "knock to the head." Athletes who suffered concussion were told to "shake it off and keep playing." As a result, little attention was paid to this injury until the late 1990s, when researchers and clinicians began focusing on concussion and its effects, primarily among athletes (e.g., M. W. Collins, Grindel, et al., 1999; M. W. Collins, Lovell, & McKeag, 1999). What these researchers found, and later reported in journals (including the *Journal of the American Medical Association*), helped put concussion on the map.

Fast-forward to 2017 and concussion is a topic of discussion in the media, medicine, politics, and even in video games. (Concussions are now "part of the game" in the popular *Madden Football* videogame franchise.) Every time we have a discussion with someone on a plane or at a party about what we do, we end up in a 15- to 20-minute discussion that includes comments and ques-tions: "Should my son quit football because of concussions?" "My daughter's unit in Afghanistan was recently exposed to an improvised explosive device, and she has had a headache for weeks." "Can those new mouth guards prevent concussion?" We would like to think these discussions occur because we are interesting conversationalists, but we are reconciled to the realization that it's the topic of concussion and its effects, known and unknown, that draws public interest.

The good news is that we know a lot more about concussion now than just a few years ago. In fact, a literature search of *PubMed* for the terms *concus-sion* or *mTBI* (mild traumatic brain injury) for the year 2016 alone returned a list of 1,174 publications. There has been a fivefold increase in the number of peer-reviewed journal articles between 1980 and 2017 (see Figure 2.1). However, this number is dwarfed by the volume of information and in some cases, misinformation, in print, Internet, and television media. In fact, a July 2017 search of *concussion* or *mTBI* in the Google search engine resulted in 145,000 returns. Concussions, from sports to the military, seem to be a con-stant lead story on the nightly news. Sometimes these stories have taken on a life of their own, as in the case of chronic traumatic encephalopathy, which has been associated (albeit with very limited empirical support) with concussions. In fact, during a 5-year period between 2010 and 2014, when a total of 66 articles on chronic traumatic encephalopathy were published in peer-reviewed journals, the *New York Times* published 290 articles on the topic (as determined through a search for *CTE* on the internal *NY Times* search engine). Numerous blogs are devoted to concussions, including the *Concussion Blog* and *Brain Blogger*, and concussion is a frequent topic on other websites such as *MomsTeam*.

Our legal system is just starting to feel the effects of the concussion wave. Concussion and its effects were the focal points of a recent lawsuit against

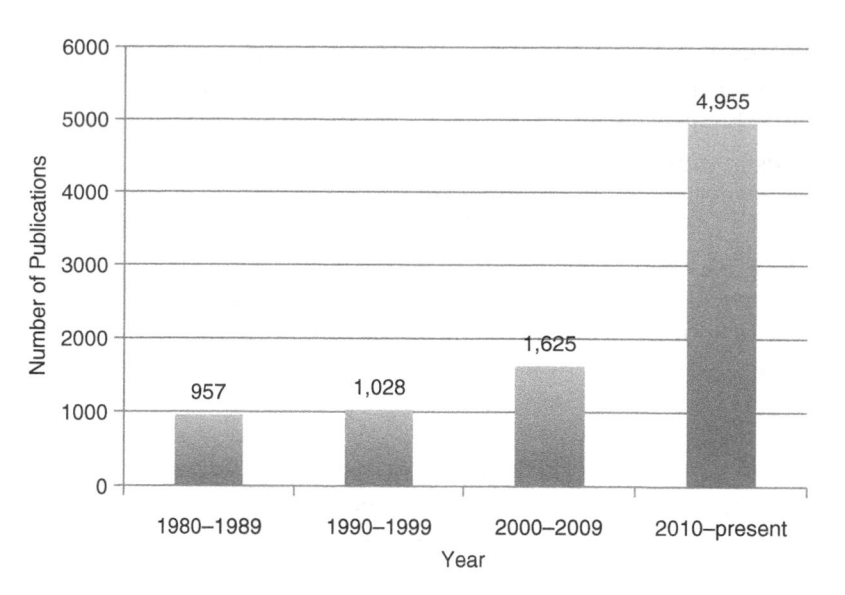

Figure 2.1. Number of publications about concussion or mild traumatic brain injury since 1980.

the National Football League involving potentially more than 20,000 former and current professional football players. These lawsuits are likely to result in hundreds of millions (if not billions) of dollars in legal fees and settlement payments. The economic impact of concussions is currently estimated by the Centers for Disease Control and Prevention (CDC; 2017) to be as high as $17 billion annually. Clearly, it is a good time to be an injury attorney specializing in head injuries.

In summary, interest in concussion is high. Some believe that the concussion pendulum has swung too far in the direction of overdiagnosis, highly conservative management of the injury, hypersensitivity on the part of parents and the media, and the assumption that all chronic conditions involving the brain (such as Alzheimer's and amyotrophic lateral sclerosis, also known as Lou Gehrig's disease) are somehow related to concussions. A brief look back at the history of this injury might provide the appropriate context for a discussion of the key concepts for this injury.

YOU'VE COME A LONG WAY BABY!
HISTORICAL CONTEXT FOR CONCUSSION

Historical references to concussions in battle or from accidents extend as far back as Ancient Greece and Egypt. In fact, *On Injuries of the Head*, an ancient predecessor to the current book, was written by Hippocrates in

400 BC. In this book, Hippocrates described methods for assessing and treating no fewer than five types of head injuries, ranging from mild to severe. In so doing, he eloquently described the challenges in assessing and treating closed head injuries, such as concussion, that persist today.

"It is not possible to recognize these varieties by sight . . . neither, indeed is it visible to the eyes when any mischief of this kind takes place" (Withington, 1928, p. 5).

Hippocrates also described the diffused nature of injury that a concussion or other head injury can cause in what he referred to as "(head) injuries at distant sites" (Withington, 1928, p. 8). He described further that these injuries could be a challenge to assess and treat, as the effects do not necessarily correspond to the location of the injury. The resemblance of these challenges from 400 BC to those facing clinicians today is uncanny. Such examples provide more evidence that one should always glance back before moving forward.

Although the term *concussion* was not used in its current form until the 1500s AD (P. R. McCrory & Berkovic, 2001), early descriptions of the injury are consistent with modern day concepts (Seymour, 2013). In fact, loss of consciousness was the predominant clinical symptom included in these early descriptions (P. R. McCrory & Berkovic, 2001), and it remains a critical symptom in current concussion grading scales. Other symptoms described in these historical accounts included visual problems, imbalance, and speech and hearing loss. Not surprisingly, these early characterizations of concussion focused on the most observable signs and symptoms. One area of agreement in descriptions of concussion since the 900s AD is in the transient nature of the injury (P. R. McCrory & Berkovic, 2001). In short, concussions were viewed as different from severe brain injuries in that their effects were not permanent.

WHAT'S IN A NAME? DEFINING *CONCUSSION*

The term *concussion* originates from the Latin *concutere*, which literally translates to "shake violently," "disturb," or "strike together" (P. R. McCrory & Berkovic, 2001). You have to hand it to the Romans for providing a clear and straightforward term that is still relevant today. Of course, the definition for concussion has evolved over time, but not as much as one might think. In fact, with a few exceptions, concussion definitions may have become less clear and more complicated over time. This complication of definitions tends to occur whenever experts gather to develop a consensus or researchers are involved in the process of defining a term.

A summary of concussion definitions from a variety of organizations is provided in Table 2.1. Many of the definitions refer to similar characteristics,

TABLE 2.1
Definitions of Concussion From the Literature

Date	Study authors	Group	Definition
2003	Parmet, Lynm, and Glass	American Medical Association	An injury to the brain caused by a blow to the head that results in temporary loss of normal brain function.
2010	Halstead, Walter, and the Council on Sports Medicine and Fitness	American Academy of Pediatrics	A rapid onset of short-lived impairment of neurologic function that resolves spontaneously.
2011	American College of Sports Medicine	American College of Sports Medicine	An injury to the brain where force causes the brain to move within the skull.
2013	Giza et al.	American Academy of Neurology	A clinical syndrome of biomechanically induced alteration of brain function, typically affecting memory and orientation, which may involve loss of consciousness.
2013	Harmon et al.	American Medical Society for Sports Medicine	A traumatically induced transient disturbance of brain function and involves a complex pathophysiologic process.
2017	McCrory et al.	Berlin International Consensus Statement	A traumatic brain injury induced by biomechanical forces. Several common features that may be utilized in clinically defining the nature of a concussive head injury . . . (followed by bulleted list of common features).
2016	NCAA Sport Science Institute	National Collegiate Athletic Association	A change in brain function following a force to the head, which may be accompanied by temporary loss of consciousness, but is identified in awake individuals, with measures of neurologic and cognitive dysfunction.
2014	Broglio et al.	National Athletic Trainers' Association	Traumatic-induced alteration in mental status that may or may not involve a loss of consciousness.
2014	Sarmiento, Hoffman, Dmitrovsky, and Lee	Centers for Disease Control and Prevention	A type of mild traumatic brain injury caused by a bump, blow, or jolt to the head or body that can change the way the brain normally works.
2015	Choe and Giza	Seminars in Neurology	An injury to the head as a result of blunt trauma or acceleration or deceleration forces that result in one or more of the following conditions: any period of observed or self-reported: transient confusion, disorientation, or impaired consciousness; dysfunction of memory around the time of injury; or loss of consciousness lasting less than 30 minutes.

such as the forces that cause a concussion, changes to brain function that follow a concussion, and the transient nature of the effects of the injury. Nevertheless, there is significant variation among them: the American Academy of Pediatrics definition is less clear and more open to interpretation than some definitions; the American College of Sports Medicine focuses on specific information such as the biomechanical aspects of concussion; the CDC definition is simplistic, whereas the National Collegiate Athletic Association and Seminars in Neurology definitions are more complex. Because the constituents as well as the politics and interests of each organization drive the focus and content of these definitions, no single agreed-upon definition for this injury exists. The closest to a consensus definition is the Berlin International Consensus Statement, which represents a diverse group of health care professionals and sports organizations (P. McCrory et al., 2017).

Researchers and clinicians often refer to a concussion using other terminology. Concussions are often referred to as *mild traumatic brain injuries* (mild TBI or mTBI). However, there is nothing "mild" about a TBI, so this term is somewhat of a misnomer or oxymoron. In fact, the use of the term *mild TBI* is in many ways analogous to the definition of oxymoron itself, which means dull and sharp simultaneously. That said, the term *mild TBI* is still commonly used in the literature, especially in military and hospital-based populations. The CDC definition also uses the term *mild TBI* (see Table 2.1). Concussion or mild TBI represents the beginning of the brain injury severity spectrum that also includes moderate TBI in the middle and severe TBI at the extreme end. The majority of brain injuries occur on the mild side of the spectrum, with very few moderate and severe TBIs. In fact, it is estimated that 80% to 90% of all brain injuries are concussions (Saatman et al., 2008). In the United States, about 3.8 million patients require concussion care each year (Langlois, Rutland-Brown, & Wald, 2006), which makes concussion one of the fastest growing subspecializations in the field of psychology. (In this book, we use the term *concussion* rather than *mild TBI*.)

MECHANICS OF CONCUSSION

If you have ever watched sports on TV, you have probably seen the "big hits" between opposing players and then cringed as you watched the impact. The wide receiver who is lifted off his feet and lands flat on his back following a tackle from an opposing linebacker is one example of this sort of hit. Another example is the boxer who takes an uppercut to the chin that contorts his face and violently rotates his head and neck or the ice hockey player who is cross-checked so hard that he goes flying at high speed into the boards. Each of these examples involves substantial biomechanical forces acting on the skull and brain (referred to as *accelerations*). Two primary types of accelerations result in a concussion: (a) *linear* accelerations, which are accelerations involving a single direction and are measured in g-forces (with 1 g = the force of gravity acting on earth); and (b) *rotational* or *angular* accelerations, which represent the rate of change in the velocity of a rotating body and are measured in radians per second^2 (with 1 rad/s^2 = 572 revolutions per minute). Examples of forces that relate to linear accelerations are provided in Figure 2.2.

High school and college football players are reported to experience between 520 and 652 head traumas over the course of a season (Broglio, Eckner, & Kutcher, 2012; Broglio, Eckner, et al., 2011; Schnebel, Gwin, Anderson, & Gatlin, 2007). A majority (75%) of head impacts are considered to be far below (< 30 g) the levels of concussive impacts (Broglio, Eckner, & Kutcher, 2012). However, a concussion can occur at levels lower than 30 g and higher than 90 g, numbers that have been tossed around in the literature and media as "concussive thresholds." Despite considerable debate, there is little support for a conclusive concussive impact level or threshold. Several manufacturers have capitalized on the desire for a "red light/green light" answer to concussion mechanics; however, the research to date has provided mixed support for a biomechanical threshold. In fact, currently, accelerometers or head impact

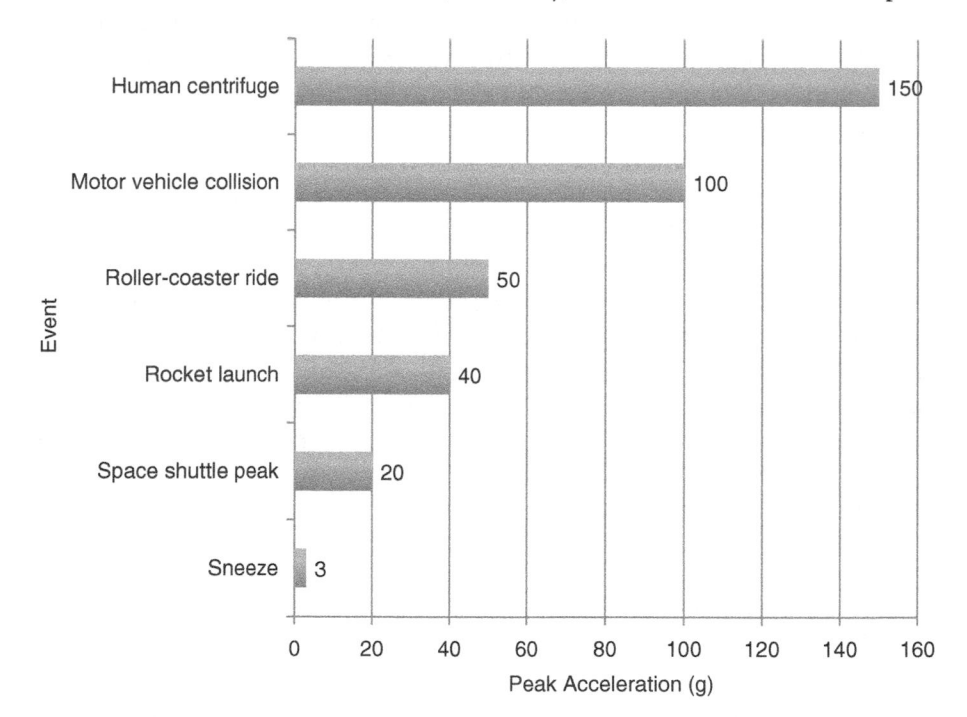

Figure 2.2. Common events that result in a variety of peak linear acceleration levels (g). Data drawn from The Physics Hypertext website (http://physics.info/acceleration/).

telemetry research has established a wide range of mean head impact thresholds; peak linear accelerations from 70 g to 102.8 g and angular accelerations from 5311.6 rad/s/s to 6111.4 rad/s/s (Broglio et al., 2009; Broglio, Eckner, et al., 2011; Broglio, Eckner, & Kutcher, 2012; Broglio, Schnebel, et al., 2010; Eckner, Sabin, Kutcher, & Broglio, 2011; Guskiewicz et al., 2007; Pellman, Viano, Tucker, Casson, & Committee on Mild Traumatic Brain Injury, 2003). To the contrary, Guskiewicz and colleagues have suggested that a single impact may not result in immediate symptoms of a concussion or subsequent balance or cognitive deficits, which supports the position that no rigid threshold for concussion can be set.

Although the biomechanical forces that result in concussion are important to our understanding of this injury and warrant additional research, our efforts may be better served focusing on the risk factors that lead certain individuals to have concussions, even at lower accelerations. Perhaps more important, we should examine which factors might protect certain individuals from the immediate effects of concussion, thereby sparing them from acute injury but perhaps leaving them prone to long-term sequelae from repeated impacts to the brain. This framework for research based on resiliency to disease (in this case injury) has yet to be used by concussion researchers. Such an approach is warranted if we want to learn why one individual can be exposed to a 150 g linear acceleration to the head and not have a concussion, whereas another individual can be exposed to a 30 g linear acceleration and have a concussion.

Another way to conceptualize the forces that result in a concussion is to think of the brain as contained inside a protective layer of cerebral spinal fluid that cushions it like an egg white cushions the egg yolk. Imagine that the skull represents the eggshell, and our picture is complete. Now imagine that someone violently shakes the egg, but instead of a nice smooth eggshell, the brain is encased in the skull with its bony protuberances that rake across the brain as it moves inside the skull. As a result, axons are stretched and may be torn from movement within the skull, resulting in diffuse axonal injury. More important, these forces acting on the brain set in motion a series of pathophysiological events that manifest as the symptoms and impairment of this injury.

PATHOPHYSIOLOGY OF CONCUSSION: THE NEUROMETABOLIC CASCADE

Typically, the healthy brain operates in a very efficient manner, requiring little energy to perform tasks. However, following injury such as a concussion, the brain becomes inefficient. Essentially, it goes from being a hybrid or electric car that requires little fuel to operate to being a large truck that requires a copious amount of fuel just to get moving. At a cellular level, the brain is in a state of crisis immediately following concussion because of an imbalance in energy demand and available resources. In short, the brain is starved for energy at a time when it desperately needs energy to start repairing itself.

Two primary events influence this process: (a) an efflux of potassium (K^+) ions outside of the cell and (b) an influx of calcium (Ca^{2+}) into the cell. These ionic shifts together with disrupted cerebral metabolism and impaired connectivity and communication result in temporary neuronal dysfunction (see Figure 2.3). This process is referred to as the *neurometabolic cascade* and is most pronounced in the first few hours and days following a concussion (Giza & Hovda, 2001, 2014). It is also during this time immediately following a concussion that the injured brain is most vulnerable to subsequent injuries (Giza & Hovda, 2014; P. McCrory et al., 2013). This period of increased vulnerability is particularly problematic for younger individuals.

BEFORE a concussion...

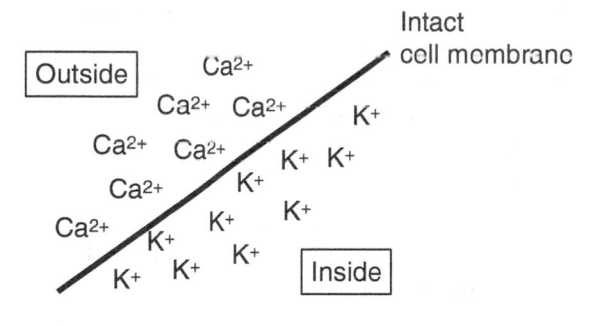

AFTER a concussion...

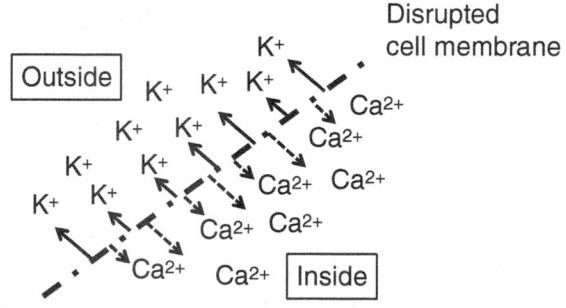

Figure 2.3. The neurometabolic cascade of concussion. Ca^2 = calcium; K = potassium.

VULNERABLE POSTINJURY PERIOD
AND SECOND IMPACT SYNDROME

Subsequent injury in this vulnerable period may lead to longer recovery (Elbin, Sufrinko, Schatz, French, Henry, et al., 2016) or potentially catastrophic injury such as second impact syndrome (SIS), which appears to affect only younger (i.e., children and young adults) brains (McLendon, Kralik, Grayson, & Golomb, 2016). Just as running on a sprained ankle can adversely affect recovery, so too can "running" on a "sprained brain." In fact, any activity (such as work, schoolwork, intense play, or even reading) that increases the demands on the injured brain may exacerbate and prolong the effects of a concussion. More specifically, both animal studies involving mice and rats (Giza, Griesbach, & Hovda, 2005; Griesbach, Hovda, Molteni, Wu, & Gomez-Pinilla, 2004; Ip, Giza, Griesbach, & Hovda, 2002) and research involving humans (N. J. Brown et al., 2014; Majerske et al., 2008) have shown that taxing the brain during the vulnerable period immediately following a concussion is a bad idea. In rare instances, this stress on the brain can even lead to death in younger individuals (typically < 18 years) from SIS (Cantu, 1992, 1998; Cantu & Gean, 2010; Cantu & Voy, 1995).

In SIS, it is theorized that when an individual with a currently symptomatic concussion incurs another blow to the head during the period of vulnerability, the result might be massive cerebral edema and bleeding inside the brain. Even seemingly mild blows to the head, particularly in individuals under the age of 18 years, typically result in mortality or long-term morbidity (McLendon et al., 2016). With SIS, an individual who is still experiencing postconcussion symptoms returns to sport (and nearly all examples of SIS have involved athletes) or some other activity and incurs a second, often innocuous-looking impact, the result may be rapid cerebral edema and in many cases death (Cantu, 1992; Cantu & Gean, 2010). Those few who survive never fully recover their neurological function and often find themselves in a coma as a result of these avoidable injuries.

Thankfully, the odds of SIS, although unknown, appear to be low; only 35 cases were identified in sport during a 13-year period between 1980 and 1993 (Bey & Ostick, 2009). However, more recently, researchers have suggested that SIS is even more rare than previously thought; a reexamination of the literature reveals that only 17 patient cases have sufficient evidence for SIS (McLendon et al., 2016). One thing is certain: You cannot get SIS without a second impact to the head during the vulnerable period following a concussion. In short, children and adolescents who have a concussion should avoid at all costs a second impact during the vulnerable periods immediately following injury (P. McCrory, Davis, & Makdissi, 2012).

DIFFUSE AXONAL INJURY

Another component of the underlying pathophysiology of concussion is diffuse axonal injury (DAI), which involves damage to axons that help the brain communicate and function. Think of the brain as having trillions of highways that connect its different regions and help them communicate with each other. These connections or highways involve white matter. Damage to the white matter tracts following concussion has been reported by researchers using diffusion tensor imaging (DTI; Babcock, Yuan, Leach, Nash, & Wade, 2015; Lange et al., 2015). Using magnetic resonance imaging technology, DTI allows us to "see" damage to regions of white matter (i.e., DAI) in the brain by visualizing the flow of water. However, the relevance of this damage to functional impairment is not well understood. Moreover, researchers have reported both increases (good: e.g., Arfanakis et al., 2002) and decreases (bad: e.g., Bazarian et al., 2007) in *fractional anisotropy* (FA), the directionality of water flow in the brain (which may be dependent on time since injury).

We recently conducted research involving both DTI and a new method for imaging white matter track damage referred to as *high-definition fiber tracking* (HDFT). While DTI allows us to see the amount and location of white matter damage, HDFT allows us to see the connection between damaged tracks or connections of white matter in the brain. In short, it lets us see which highways are damaged. Using DTI and HDFT, we imaged athletes at 1 to 14 days postinjury and again when they were cleared to return to full activity (i.e., recovered). What we found was compelling. There was decreased FA in the thalamus, which is considered a crossroads for sensory communication between the brain and body. The decreases in FA in this superhighway for sensory communication in the brain were correlated with deficits on vestibular, oculomotor, and neurocognitive tests. The HDFT findings suggested that there was damage to the corticospinal track, which represents the connection between the cortex and spinal cord and is associated with motor control and movement, that appeared to repair itself in those subjects who recovered faster. Moving forward, this emerging imaging technique may allow us to better "see" damage in the brain, track recovery, and communicate these findings in a meaningful way to patients.

CEREBROVASCULAR EFFECTS ASSOCIATED WITH CONCUSSION

In addition to the neurometabolic cascade described above, the brain experiences cerebrovascular dysautoregulation immediately following a concussion that further exacerbates the effects of this injury. Specifically, cerebral blood flow is reduced because of vasoconstriction, resulting in less oxygen and less glucose for the injured brain. Researchers have reported that these cerebrovascular changes correspond to concussion and also recover in conjunction with clinical symptoms (Meier et al., 2015). We recently reported that blood flow in concussed athletes was reduced during cognitive tasks (Kontos et al., 2014). We found that concussed individuals were less efficient when performing the same tasks as healthy controls. Moreover, this inefficiency was associated with worse cognitive performance on a computerized neurocognitive test battery called the Immediate Post-Concussion Assessment and Cognitive Test (ImPACT Applications, Inc., San Diego, California), suggesting that compromised blood flow may influence impairment following concussion.

In conclusion, the pathophysiological response following a concussion may involve neurometabolic and cerebrovascular changes, as well as DAI. These changes begin immediately following a concussion and may last several days (longer in children), during which time the brain is particularly vulnerable to additional injury and in rare circumstances to potential catastrophic outcome from SIS. As such, the early identification and management of concussion is critical to minimizing the effects of this injury. Recognizing the signs and symptoms of this injury is important to help identify and manage individuals with a concussion.

SIGNS AND SYMPTOMS OF CONCUSSION

The signs and symptoms of concussion run the gamut from confusion and memory problems to dizziness and nausea; individuals may present with many or just a few signs and symptoms. At this point in the discussion, it is important to define the terms we will be using. *Signs* are observable indications of a concussion; *symptoms* are self-reported interpretations of subjective states or feeling following injury. For example, disorientation is a sign of concussion, whereas headache is a symptom. Both signs and symptoms are important in identifying and assessing the severity of the injury.

Signs

The signs of concussion are important to recognize, because they provide some of the first indicators that a concussion has indeed occurred. Exhibit 2.1 summarizes the common signs of this injury and signs that warrant immediate medical attention. Traditionally, the hallmark sign of concussion was loss of consciousness (LOC), or being "knocked out." LOC can be brief, lasting seconds to a minute, or it can be prolonged (up to 20 minutes) following a concussion. Any individual with LOC lasting longer than 20 minutes is considered

EXHIBIT 2.1
Common Signs of Concussion and Emergent Symptoms
That Warrant Immediate Attention

Commons sign of concussion	Emergent symptoms that warrant immediate medical attention
Loss of consciousness < 30 seconds	Loss of consciousness > 30 seconds
Posttraumatic amnesia < 24 hours	Repeated vomiting
Disorientation	Worsening symptoms
Confusion	Rapid change in mental status
Vomiting	Headache that worsen or moves around
Imbalance	Severe irritability
Dizziness	Sudden behavior change
Nausea	Slurred, slowed or confused speech
Numbness	Seizure
Tingling	Problems with motor coordination
Vision problems (blurry, double vision)	Dilated or unequal pupils

to have a moderate or severe TBI, rather than a concussion. In fact, 20 years ago, LOC was essential to a diagnosis of concussion. Most grading scales that were developed to assess the severity of this injury (e.g., Kelly, 2001) were predicated on the presence or absence of LOC. However, using LOC as the basis for a diagnosis of concussion resulted in many missed injuries. In fact, only about 10% of all concussions involve brief LOC (Guskiewicz, Weaver, Padua, & Garrett, 2000), which means that about 90% of what we now know were concussions were missed using the old grading scales.

Another sign of concussion is posttraumatic amnesia (PTA), which can be either retrograde (memory of events before the injury) or anterograde (memory of events after the injury). Some researchers have suggested that PTA is an important predictor of poor outcomes following a concussion, including worse impairment and prolonged recovery time (M. W. Collins et al., 2003). Disorientation and confusion, together with brief LOC (< 30 seconds) and posttraumatic amnesia (< 24 hours), are widely considered to be the key signs of a concussion. Evidence of disorientation and confusion following a concussion might include uncertainty of the current place, time, and context of events. After a concussion, an individual might repeat answers to questions already asked or ask for questions to be repeated. Sometimes disorientation and confusion are subtle, whereas other times they are more obvious. For example, in the 2014 World Cup final, German defender Christoph Kramer was concussed in a collision with an opponent. Unfortunately, he was not removed from the field immediately following his injury (we could write a whole other chapter on why he was not removed, but we will leave that for the second edition!), and about 15 minutes later apparently went up to the referee and asked, "Where am I? Is this the (World Cup) final?"—a clear sign of disorientation.

Additional signs of this injury might include problems with motor coordination, imbalance, and difficulty following directions. Other less common but more overt signs of concussion include nausea and vomiting, which often occur concurrently. Another overt but infrequent sign is numbness or tingling. It is important to note that certain signs of concussion may be indicative of more serious brain injury and warrant immediate emergency medical care (see Exhibit 2.1).

Symptoms

Concussion symptoms are both varied and individualized. Symptoms are determined by a variety of factors, including the nature (e.g., mechanism location, biomechanical forces) of the injury as well as preinjury risk factors such as age, sex, concussion history, and migraine history. As such, it is important to assess a variety of symptoms with this injury. Consequently, between 20 and 25 symptoms typically accompany this injury and need to be considered by clinicians. Some symptoms occur more frequently than others, whereas some symptoms occur only occasionally following concussion. Not surprisingly, headache is the most common symptom of a concussion. In fact, in a study we conducted involving more than 1,400 patients during the first week following a concussion, approximately 75% reported headache (Kontos, Elbin, et al., 2012; see Table 2.2). Other common symptoms included difficulty concentrating, fatigue, drowsiness, and dizziness. Less common symptoms that occurred in fewer than 40% of concussions included balance and memory problems. Also among the least common symptoms following a concussion are vomiting and numbness/tingling occurring in 7% and 11% of concussions, respectively. It is important to note that although certain types of symptoms may occur less frequently, such as sleep-related and affective symptoms, they may play a significant role in recovery time and related outcomes following concussion.

HOW TO CONCEPTUALIZE AND PRIORITIZE SYMPTOMS: TIMING IS EVERYTHING

Although each concussion is individualized, symptom patterns can be detected. Some of these patterns are temporal in nature, whereas others involve different groups or categories of symptom clusters (similar symptoms that "hang" together in logical groups). The type of symptom clusters that occur is influenced by time since injury. In other words, symptoms occur in

TABLE 2.2
Frequency of Commonly Reported Symptoms
During the First Week After a Concussion

Frequency	Symptoms	% reporting
# 1	Headache	75
# 2	Difficulty concentrating	57
# 3	Fatigue	52
# 4	Drowsiness	51
# 5	Dizziness	49
# 6	Feeling mentally "foggy"	47
# 7	Feeling slowed down	46
# 8	Sensitivity to light	45
# 9 (tie)	Balance problems	39
# 9 (tie)	Difficulty remembering	39
# 11	Sensitivity to noise	37
# 12	Trouble falling asleep	34
# 13	Nausea	33
# 14	Irritability	29
# 15	Visual problems	25
# 16	Sleeping more than usual	23
# 17	Sleeping less than usual	22
# 18	Nervousness	18
# 19	Feeling more emotional	17
# 20	Sadness	16
# 21	Numbness or tingling	11
# 22	Vomiting	7

Note. N = 1,438.

different patterns based on the time since injury. Therefore, it is important for clinicians and researchers to understand these patterns in order to make sense of presenting symptomatology and changes in symptoms over time.

When treating concussion, clinicians must be mindful of time since injury, which is classified as *acute, subacute,* or *chronic.* There is some debate regarding the length of each clinical time period following a concussion. Most of the debate centers on the acute period, during which the brain is most vulnerable to additional injury. Some clinicians and researchers believe the acute time period only extends to the first 72 hours postinjury; see, for example, the recent Sports Concussion Common Data Elements categories of the National Institute for Neurological Disorders and Stroke. Others believe that the acute time period spans the time from injury through the first week following injury. Age and other risk factors may also play a role in the nature of these time periods; some clinicians believe that this time period is extended up to a week for younger individuals following a concussion, particularly for adolescents. The recent child-specific recommendations from the Concussion in Sport Group meeting in Berlin provide an excellent resource on the effects of age on recovery and clinical outcomes (Davis et al., 2017). Regardless, during the acute period, the brain is highly vulnerable to additional injury and symptoms tend to be more global in nature (Kontos, Elbin, et al., 2012). During this early time period, pediatric and primary care physicians typically provide clinical care. In sports, athletic trainers and sport medicine physicians often provide initial care. In more severe concussions, where more serious intracranial pathology (e.g., subdural hematoma) is possible or suspected, patients may seek care in an emergency department or urgent care clinic.

The subacute time period occurs immediately following the acute time period, that is, approximately 3 to 5 days postinjury, and it lasts up to 3 months. Individuals during the subacute time period begin to have more distinct symptom profiles (see below). Most individuals will recover from a concussion during this time period, typically within the first month postinjury (Henry, Elbin, Collins, Marchetti, & Kontos, 2016; P. McCrory et al., 2013). The subacute time period is also when most patients seek specialized care for their injury. In general, research studies on concussion are limited to the first month or so after the injury. However, little research exists on what transpires during the later subacute time period between 1 and 3 months. Based on the management of the injury, this period is likely critical to the development of chronic concussion symptoms, which are often referred to as postconcussion syndrome or symptoms (P. McCrory et al., 2013).

The chronic time period is defined as 3 months or more following injury and is characterized by lingering symptoms and impairment. Patients in this time period are among the most challenging to manage because it is difficult for clinicians to discern between injury-related and psychological symptoms (Iverson, 2006). Consequently, during the chronic time period, a variety of specialized clinicians may be involved in the care of patients, including clinical and neuropsychologists, neurologists, vestibular and physical therapists, and vision specialists, to name a few.

Clinicians often aggregate similar symptoms into groups or clusters (also known as factors) that represent some clinically meaningful construct. For example, clinicians who specialize in the treatment of patients with anxiety disorders have traditionally grouped symptoms into categories such as physical or somatic, emotional, and behavioral. This approach is intuitive to both clinicians and patients and can also help to inform better clinical conceptualization and direct more effective assessment, management and treatment strategies. For example, a concussed athlete presenting predominately with cognitive symptoms (e.g., difficulty concentrating, memory problems) may benefit from different management and treatment programs when compared with an individual with a postinjury migraine presentation or affective presentation. Specific clinical management approaches (e.g., specific academic accommodations), treatment strategies (e.g., neurostimulant vs. preventative migraine medication), and rehabilitation plans (e.g., exertional activity vs. rest) may be determined by these symptom factors. Moreover, proper establishment of concussion symptom factors may provide an appropriate foundation to research different subtypes of concussive injury and more targeted outcome studies aimed at treatment and rehabilitation.

Symptom Factors

Clinicians specializing in treating concussion have categorized concussion-related symptoms into two, three, or four factors (Herrmann et al., 2009; Piland, Motl, Ferrara, & Peterson, 2003; Piland, Motl, Guskiewicz, McCrea, & Ferrara, 2006). These factors are typically categorized as *affective/emotional*, *cognitive*, *sleep-related*, or *physical/somatic*. Although these symptom factor structures are predicated on clinical meaning, they are supported by factor analytic statistical methods. Figure 2.4 shows one of these symptom factor structures using the symptom items from the Post-Concussion Symptom Scale (PCSS) as discussed in the Pardini et al. (2004) study. We noticed that all of the

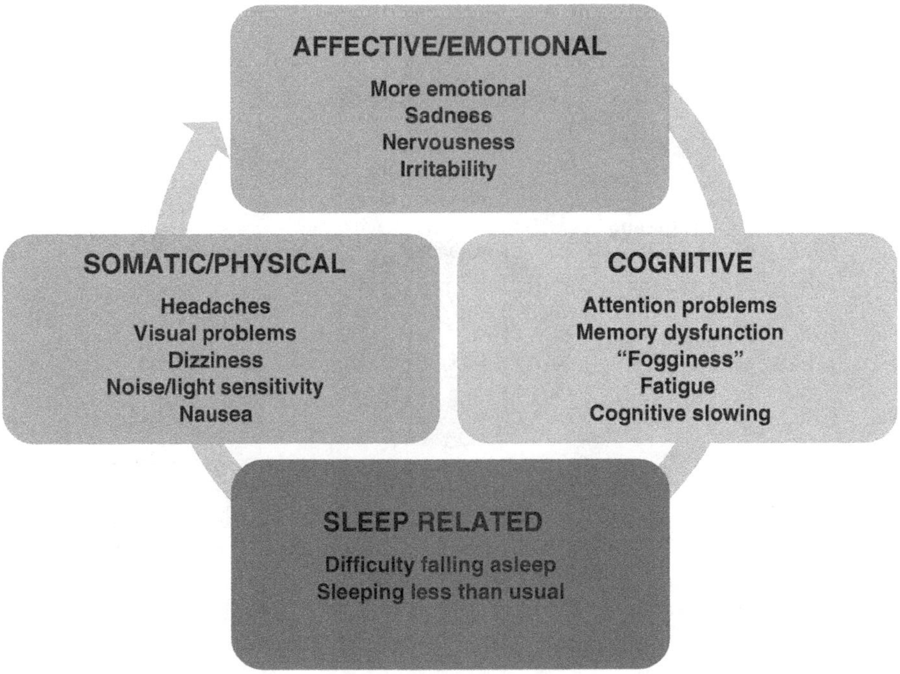

Figure 2.4. Common symptom factors including affective/emotional, somatic/physical, cognitive, and sleep-related factors 1 or more weeks after concussion.

previous studies on symptom factors had a common feature: fairly lengthy time periods since injury ranging from several weeks to several months. None of the studies focused on the patients during the first week postinjury specifically. However, the nature of symptoms during this critical time period for assessing and beginning the management of this injury was largely unknown. Hence, we conducted a study to see what symptoms look like during that first week following injury.

We examined the symptoms of 1,438 athletes with a concussion from a 5-year time period between 2006 and 2011. We looked at symptom factors at 1 week postconcussion and also compared age and sex cohorts. The findings supported a "global" symptom factor that comprised what we termed *cognitive-fatigue-migraine* symptoms (see Figure 2.5; Kontos, Elbin, et al., 2012). Additional, small affective, sleep, and somatic factors were also supported, but they were not very strong. Not surprisingly, females reported more symptoms (particularly affective symptoms) than males. College-aged athletes reported more sleep symptoms postinjury than high school athletes. However, despite these differences, the factor structures remained stable across age and sex groups. Based on our findings, we believe that symptoms during the first week

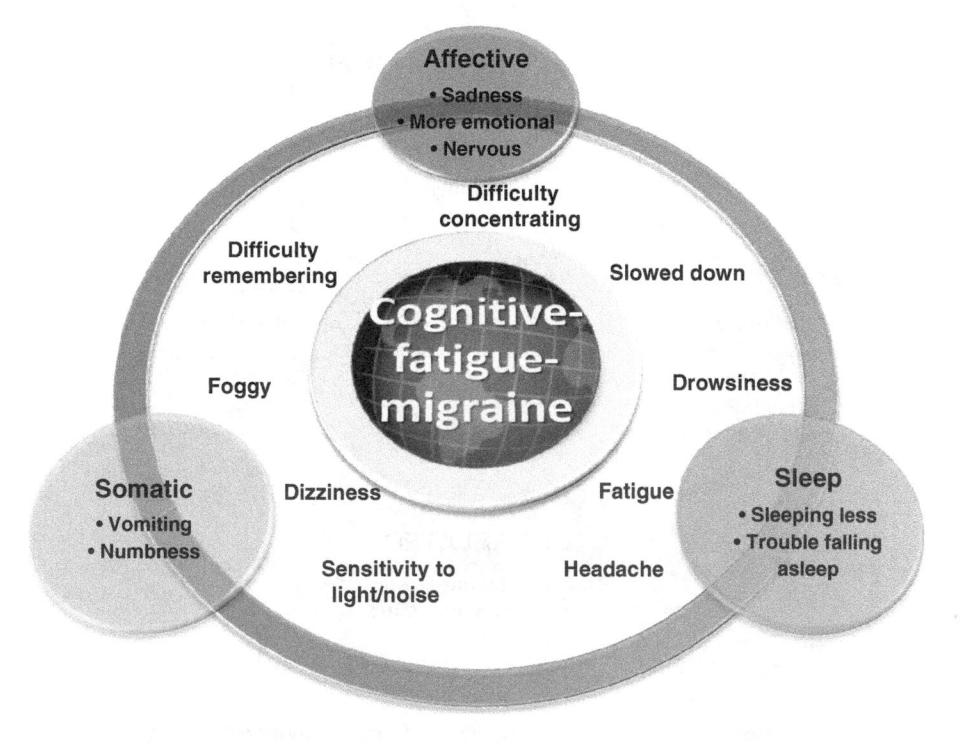

Figure 2.5. Concussion symptom factors during the first week after an injury.

postinjury are broad and cover multiple domains. In contrast, for patients with prolonged recoveries, as the time from injury increases, the symptoms cluster into more distinct factors as reported previously in the literature (Pardini et al., 2004). Given the global nature of symptoms in the first few days postinjury, more conservative management strategies may be warranted.

Baseline Symptoms Matter

The assessment of concussion symptoms is a cornerstone to assessing individuals with this injury (P. McCrory et al., 2013). However, concussion symptoms are typically assessed only at postinjury time intervals. In other words, clinicians usually do not know a patient's preinjury or baseline level of symptoms. Researchers have reported that baseline levels of concussion-related symptoms among healthy individuals vary considerably, with some individuals reporting no symptoms at baseline and others reporting high levels (Iverson & Lange, 2003). Several explanations have been posited for this variability in symptoms among healthy individuals, including the overlap between concussion-related symptoms and symptoms from other health conditions, including fatigue, orthopedic injuries, and physical illness (Piland, Ferrara, Macciocchi, Broglio, & Gould, 2010). Many different health conditions share symptoms such as headache, fatigue, dizziness, and sleeping problems, all of which are common following a concussion.

Regardless of the origin of baseline symptoms, the assessment of post-concussion symptoms in the absence of the context of premorbid symptomatology may provide inaccurate or misleading information. It has been speculated that individuals with high levels of baseline symptoms are more likely to have higher levels of postinjury symptoms as a result of their elevated starting point (Custer et al., 2016). Therefore, we decided to see whether baseline symptoms were associated with worse symptoms following concussion. We also wanted to see whether higher symptoms at baseline might be related to cognitive impairment following injury. We compared a group of patients reporting no symptoms at baseline with another group of patients reporting high levels (i.e., total symptom severity score > 18, which is high for a healthy individual) of symptoms at baseline to determine whether the groups experienced more symptoms and worse impairment following injury. What we found was unexpected. Although the groups differed in baseline symptoms, their symptoms at 1 week following injury were essentially identical. In other words, contrary to conventional opinion, patients with higher baseline symptoms did not report higher postinjury symptoms. However, these patients did experience more significant declines in memory than those with no symptoms at baseline. Together, these findings suggest that knowing something about a patient's baseline symptoms may help clinicians identify those patients at risk for worse impairment following concussion so that they can be provided with more effective therapy/treatment for their injury.

Another thing to consider regarding baseline symptoms is that certain types of symptoms, more so than others, may set the stage for worse outcomes. One group of baseline symptoms may be particularly important to consider: sleep-related symptoms. Our research suggests that at least one third of patients report one or more sleep-related difficulties (see Table 2.2). Researchers have indicated that reduced sleep duration may adversely influence concussion outcomes, including higher symptoms following injury (McClure, Zuckerman, Kutscher, Gregory, & Solomon, 2014; Mihalik et al., 2013). However, the role of preexisting sleep-related symptoms on outcomes following concussion is less established. We examined the role of preinjury sleep difficulties (specifically trouble falling asleep or sleeping less than usual) on symptoms and impairment in a large sample of concussed patients. The results indicated that patients with preinjury sleep difficulties demonstrated greater postinjury cognitive impairment and increased symptoms compared with those who did not endorse baseline sleep difficulties. The impairments were specific to memory and reaction time, both of which are affected by disrupted sleep (Gavett, Stern, & McKee, 2011; Vedaa, West Saxvig, Wilhelmsen-Langeland, Bjorvatn, & Pallesen, 2012). In short, preexisting sleep difficulties may slow processing speed and reaction time and increase symptoms following concussion. Additionally, age may interact with sleep in its effect on concussion outcomes. Adolescents who experience concussion may be at particularly high risk for developing sleep-related symptoms from subsequent concussion because they are often sleep deprived (a function of age-related disrupted sleep schedules; Halstead, Walter, & the Council on Sports Medicine and Fitness, 2010; Jan et al., 2010), and their brains are still in development (Field, Collins, Lovell, & Maroon, 2003). Therefore, it is important for clinicians to identify athletes who are at risk for worse outcomes following a concussion because of preexisting sleep difficulties.

Different Approaches to Interpreting Symptoms

Clinicians need to consider the way in which concussion symptoms are assessed. Several approaches are used to assess symptoms following concussion, and each one provides a different perspective. The most common approach involves looking at a total severity score, wherein all of the individual symptom item scores (which typically range from 0–6, 1–5, or 0–10) are totaled to provide an overall indication of symptom severity. This approach provides a good indication of the overall severity of symptoms, but it does not address which symptoms are occurring and at which levels. Another common approach is based on the total number of symptoms being reported. For example, an individual may report 10 symptoms, which provides information on the extent of symptoms but provides little information about their overall severity.

A less common but important method is to calculate an average severity score, which involves dividing the total severity score by the number of symptoms selected on a checklist. This approach provides an assessment of the intensity across symptoms. However, if a clinician relies on only one method, important information may be missed. For example, Cyndi, who has a total symptom severity of 20, has endorsed eight symptoms ranging from headache to fatigue. However, she has endorsed dizziness as a 6 (severe), whereas the remaining seven symptoms are all rated as 2. In contrast, Brandon also has a total symptom severity score of 20, but he has endorsed only four symptoms—headache, nausea, sensitivity to light, and vision problems—all at a 5 (moderately severe). Finally, Natalie, who also has a total symptom severity score of 20, has endorsed 13 different symptoms and given each a severity rating of either 1 or 2. Each of these patients had the same total symptom severity score but very different underlying symptomatology. Therefore, it is important both to consider each of these methods when examining symptom reports and to look at each symptom individually and in combination to help direct referrals and targeted treatments. A headache with cognitive fatigue throughout the day demands a different approach to treatment than a headache with nausea and sensitivity to light.

It is also important to realize that several different methods are available for assessing symptoms and multiple sources of information provide symptom-related information. The most common source of information for symptoms is, of course, the patient. However, the patient is not always the most reliable source of information because he or she has just had a brain injury. In addition, some patients may be motivated to exaggerate symptoms (as in cases of litigation or other secondary gain) or minimize them (as in the case of an athlete who underreports symptoms in order to expedite his return to sport). Other patients may simply lack insight into their symptoms, not be very good at describing them, or attribute them to causes other than their injury. As such, it is also important to gather information about symptoms from other sources, especially family members, who are more likely to notice subtle changes in behavior, mood, and cognition. Recent research suggests that agreement between parents and kids reporting their symptoms ranges from poor to nearly perfect, which supports the importance of obtaining information regarding symptoms from several sources (Rowhani-Rahbar, Chrisman, Drescher, Schiff, & Rivara, 2016). We found that parents were comparable to children when using a closed-ended symptom report (Elbin, Knox, et al., 2016). Nonetheless, using multiple sources of information to determine symptoms will provide a more comprehensive and accurate assessment of symptoms following concussion.

Typically, symptoms are assessed using self-reported measures that patients complete on a computer or using paper and pencil. (We discuss symptom assessments in more depth in Chapter 4.) This approach involves closed-ended questions that "prompt" patients to indicate whether they have a certain symptom and if so, how severe each symptom is on a Likert-type scale. Sometimes clinicians guide the patients through an oral symptom report rather than having them complete the report on a computer or piece of paper. Other approaches used to assess symptoms include open-ended clinical interview questions, such as "Which symptoms are you currently experiencing related to your injury?" Using this approach, clinicians ask patients to describe symptoms that come to mind and then indicate a severity for each symptom they report. However, the way in which symptoms are assessed may influence the number and severity of symptoms patients report. In fact, closed-ended questions may result in inflated symptoms as a result of prompting, and open-ended questions may result in underreported symptoms. In a recent study, we reported that closed-ended, guided interview symptom reports result in significantly higher numbers of reported symptoms than do open-ended interviews (Elbin, Knox, et al., 2016). We also found that open-ended interviews result in lower symptom severity scores than do guided or prompted interviews. Clinicians should use multiple methods and be aware of the effects different methods have on reported symptoms.

RISK PROFILES FOR CONCUSSION OUTCOMES: IDENTIFYING THE "MISERABLE MINORITY"

One of the biggest challenges facing the field of concussion is identifying the key risk profiles for poor prognosis (i.e., longer recovery times, worse symptoms and impairment) following this injury. Clinicians need to be able to identify what Iverson (2006) and others referred to as the "miserable minority"—those few individuals who do not follow normal recovery trajectories following concussion. When we examine risk profiles for poor outcomes following concussion, we need to consider whether the risk profile involves something that an individual brings to the table, so to speak (e.g., age, genetic factors), or something that occurs following a concussion (e.g., certain types of signs or symptoms). The former, which are referred to as *primary factors* or *premorbid risk factors*, exist a priori to the injury and often involve demographic risk factors such as age, sex, or medical history. In contrast, *secondary risk factors* occur following a concussion (often referred to as *postinjury risk factors*). Risk profiles can also be conceptualized as either modifiable (through education, prevention, or intervention) or nonmodifiable or static (e.g., sex, age).

The Big Three: Age, Sex, Concussion History

Among the more established primary or demographic risk factors for poor outcomes following concussion are age, sex, and concussion history. Each of the major published concussion consensus statements mentions these factors as potential modifiers for concussion risk and outcomes (e.g., Giza et al., 2013; P. McCrory et al., 2013, 2017).

Age

Specifically, age is suggested to be negatively associated with outcomes: Younger (e.g., high school–aged) individuals purportedly experience worse outcomes than their older (e.g., college-aged) counterparts. One reason for this proposed relationship is the potential adverse effects of concussion on the developing brains of younger individuals (Institute of Medicine & National Research Council, 2014; Meehan, Taylor, & Proctor, 2011).

In 2003, Field and colleagues provided one of the first empirical studies to compare younger and older athletes with regard to concussion-related outcomes. Using the Hopkins verbal memory and other cognitive tasks, they reported that high school–aged athletes experienced more pronounced cognitive deficits and longer recovery time than college-aged athletes. Although this initial seminal study is often overrelied upon as a reference to support age as a risk factor for poor outcomes following concussion, subsequent studies have provided additional support for age as a risk factor. In fact, in our own research we have reported that high school athletes performed worse on memory tasks and balance than college athletes in the first few days after injury (Covassin, Elbin, Harris, Parker, & Kontos, 2012). Moreover, deficits in memory persisted longer than a week for the high school athletes, whereas balance returned to normal by this time. In general, studies have shown that adolescents are at greater risk for poor outcomes following a concussion than college-aged adults (Fazio, Lovell, Pardini, & Collins, 2007; Field et al., 2003; McCrea et al., 2013; Sim, Terryberry-Spohr, & Wilson, 2008). However, the focus in these studies has been on comparing adolescents with adults. Preadolescent children have not been considered.

Despite findings that suggest that younger age is a risk factor, this notion has begun to be challenged by some researchers. Researchers have recently challenged the perspective that younger kids are at greater risk for severe outcomes after concussion than older kids. A study by Purcell, Harvey, and Seabrook (2016) indicated that 8- to 12-year-olds experienced shorter recovery times and quicker return to activity than did 13- to 17-year-olds. This finding is one of the first to counter the notion that younger kids are more susceptible to the effects of concussion than their college-aged counterparts.

However, elementary school–aged kids were not considered in previous research. As such, it may be that age has more of a curvilinear relationship with concussion outcomes as opposed to the previously supposed linear relationship (see Figure 2.6).

This new finding also hints at the potential role of *neuroplasticity*—the brain's ability to change, reorganize, or compensate for injury, insults, or other changes to the environment or the brain's structure. It has long been recognized that younger brains are more plastic or malleable, which allows for better adaptation to injury or disease involving the brain. Exercise can positively influence neuroplasticity (e.g., Svensson, Lexell, & Deierborg, 2015) and may be an appropriate therapy at certain times for some individuals following this injury. We examine the role of more active approaches to rehabilitation from concussion (and the theory behind these approaches) in Chapter 5.

Sex

The role of sex on the risk for and effects of concussion has received a lot of attention from researchers, clinicians, and the media. During the past few years, several news stories on major networks have featured girls with concussions. One such story focused on a team on which several girls had multiple concussions during a short time period, leading to the retirement of

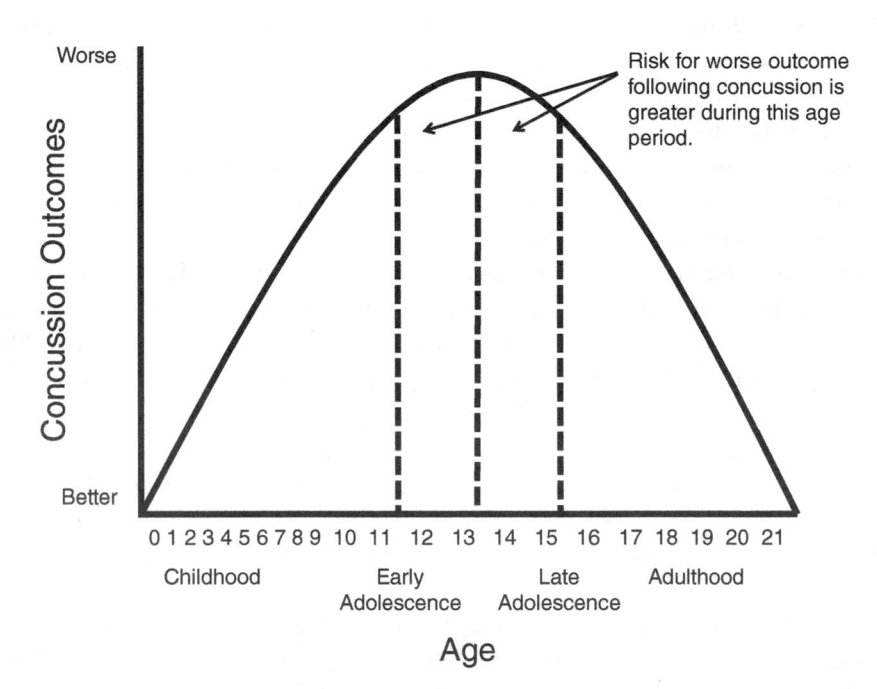

Figure 2.6. Age and concussion outcomes may be worse during early adolescence than in childhood and later adolescence and adulthood.

several players while they were still in high school. Although this example is extreme, it (and the blog comments from scared parents that followed) highlights the need to take a closer look at the role of sex on concussion risk and outcomes. It has long been suggested that females are more at risk for concussion and experience worse outcomes following this injury than their male counterparts. Researchers have reported that females are indeed at greater risk for concussion in equivalent sports and exposure levels than are males (Gessel, Fields, Collins, Dick, & Comstock, 2007; Lincoln et al., 2011). In other words, when sports like football are taken out of the equation and we compare male and female soccer, ice hockey, lacrosse or basketball players directly, we find that females in these same sports are more likely to have a concussion than males. In addition, females seem to have worse outcomes following concussion than males (Broshek et al., 2005; Covassin & Elbin, 2011; Covassin, Elbin, Harris, et al., 2012). Findings from our research indicate that females report more symptoms and perform worse on memory tasks than males following concussion (Covassin, Elbin, Harris, et al., 2012). Surprisingly, these deficits were evident in balance impairment in the first 3 days postinjury too, which is contrary to conventional wisdom that suggests that in general females are better at balance than males.

Some researchers have called into question previously reported differences between females and males in the number and severity of concussion signs and symptoms (Frommer et al., 2011). These researchers instead have suggested that females experience different types of signs and symptoms than do males, namely, more sensitivity to noise and drowsiness. Our research suggests that females are more likely to experience overall symptoms, but in particular, dizziness and vestibulo-ocular symptoms, during the first 4 weeks postinjury than males (Henry et al., 2016). These findings were supported by the results of another study of healthy collegiate athletes, in which we found that females were 3 times more likely to have vestibular and/or oculomotor impairment and symptoms at baseline than males (Kontos, Sufrinko, Elbin, Puskar, & Collins, 2016). This finding suggests that some of the postinjury differences in symptoms may be attributable to preinjury symptoms. One of our former research fellows, an obstetric-gynecologist who studied the role of concussion on menstrual dysfunction in adolescent girls, recently reported that approximately 84% of them reported PTM-related symptoms (Snook, Henry, Sanfilippo, Zeleznik, & Kontos, 2017). Given that PTM is associated with prolonged recovery and more pronounced impairment following concussion, its prevalence in concussed females may also help to explain sex differences.

Females also appear to take longer to recover following a concussion than males. In our own study comparing boys and girls, we found that females were 2.5 times more likely to be symptomatic at 30 days postinjury than males (Henry et al., 2016). Kostyun and Hafeez (2015) reported that 42% of adolescent girls took longer than 60 days to recover, compared with only 21% of males. Females were also more likely than males to be prescribed treatment following concussion. Specifically, females were 3.6 times more likely to have academic accommodations, 8.2 times more likely to have vestibular therapy, and 4.2 times more likely to be prescribed medications than males. Similarly, Henry et al. (2016) recently reported that males were 2.5 times more likely to be symptom free at 4 weeks postconcussion than females. Some of the sex differences in recovery may be related to perceptions, as we reported in a study of adolescents following concussion (Sandel, Lovell, Kegel, Collins, & Kontos, 2013). Specifically, females seem to focus more on symptoms, especially somatic, cognitive and sleep-related symptoms, in determining recovery, whereas males focus on cognitive and other impairments in addition to all types of symptoms. However, males perceive their recovery as occurring earlier than females, which seems to support the notion that females experience prolonged symptoms. (It is also possible that males are simply inaccurate in their perceptions of recovery.)

Several explanations have been posited to explain sex differences for risk and outcomes following concussion, including hormonal influences (Emerson, Headrick, & Vink, 1993); cerebrovascular differences (de Courten-Myers, 1999; Esposito, Van Horn, Weinberger, & Berman, 1996); weak neck and support muscles (Tierney et al., 2005); and other anatomical differences, such as longer cervical spine segments (Barth, Freeman, Broshek, & Varney, 2001) and body size or mass (Covassin, Elbin, Bleecker, Lipchik, & Kontos, 2013). With regard to hormonal differences, researchers have suggested that both estrogen and progesterone may act as neuroprotective factors for brain injury (through antioxidant and antiinflammatory effects, respectively; Roof & Hall, 2000). However, these neuroprotective effects may be mediated by base levels of these hormones. In other words, the effects may be different in males and females, as reported in the animal model research of Emerson and colleagues. Females may also have a higher base rate of cerebrovascular and neurometabolic functioning that is more susceptible to the neurometabolic cascade that accompanies concussion (Broshek et al., 2005). In short, female brains may have "farther to fall" after a concussion than males. The argument for sex differences in concussion outcomes resulting from differences in neck strength, with females having weaker neck musculature in general; are intuitive but have limited empirical support other than a study by C. L. Collins et al. (2014). In addition, the relationship of neck musculature to concussion is likely moderated by joint and skeletal structure, reaction time, anticipatory timing, and other factors.

Researchers have also suggested that body mass index (BMI) differences may account for sex differences in concussion outcomes. Our research group has hypothesized that lower BMI might be related to lower neck strength

(Colvin et al., 2009). Some researchers have supported this contention, finding that lower BMI is associated with higher risk of concussion (Schulz et al., 2004). However, in a study we conducted that controlled for BMI, we found that females still reported more symptoms and performed worse on memory than did males following concussion (Covassin, Elbin, Bleecker, Lipchik, & Kontos, 2013). Other explanations that may account for differences (at least in reported symptoms) suggest that females may be more forthright and honest, may have better insight, or may experience more symptoms in general that overlap with concussion symptoms (Covassin, Elbin, Larson, & Kontos, 2012). In addition, males may be habituated to ignore symptoms and "play through pain," resulting in lower reported symptoms (Kontos & Elbin, 2016).

Concussion History

With regard to concussion history, the picture is less clear. Some researchers have intimated that a history of one or two previous concussions increases the likelihood for additional injuries and worse impairment and symptoms following injury (e.g., Covassin, Stearne, & Elbin, 2008). However, other researchers have suggested that for a concussion history to have any relevance, an individual must have sustained at least three or more previous injuries (the "magic number" of previous concussions; e.g., Iverson, Gaetz, Lovell, & Collins, 2004). In fact, Quigley's Rule, which states that if an athlete has had three or more previous concussions they must be retired from sports, is predicated on this notion. As a result of this arbitrary threshold for previous concussions, undoubtedly many athletes were forced to retire from sport with little empirical evidence that this decision was necessary or beneficial. Although the motivation behind Quigley's Rule was well intended, many athletes are able to return following a third, fourth, fifth, or even more concussions, assuming the injuries were properly treated. Additionally, a simple concussion history that focuses on numbers of previous injuries fails to take into account the time since injury. In other words, the key question may be, "Was the previous concussion recent (i.e., within the past month or two) or was it distant (i.e., several months to years in the past)?" However, to date, there is no research on time since injury of previous concussions on risk of future injuries and outcomes of current injuries.

Currie, Comstock, Fields, and Cantu (2017) did compare patients with initial and recurrent (i.e., patients with a concussion history) concussions and found that they did not differ with regard to outcomes. This finding suggests that a simple assessment of yes–no for concussion history may not matter much with regard to recovery. Another critical component influencing the role of concussion history on subsequent risk and outcomes is whether the previous injury was properly managed or treated prior to return to activity. In short, if an individual is not properly healed from a previous injury, the effects of a "second" injury—which is really an extension of the first, mismanaged concussion—then the negative effect of the previous injury will be magnified. As such, it is critical to properly manage, treat, and monitor recovery from this injury to ensure an individual's concussion is not exacerbated by subsequent injury to the brain.

Emerging Risk Profiles

In addition to the more established risk factors discussed in the preceding section, certain emerging primary and secondary risk factors prior to a concussion or particular signs and symptoms following a concussion may result in a more severe injury and warrant additional attention from clinicians. Although the empirical evidence for these emerging risk factors is limited, we believe they warrant discussion; from a clinical perspective, these factors seem to influence outcomes and should be considered in the assessment and treatment of patients with this injury. We have also included a brief discussion of genetic risk factors.

Emerging Primary Risk Factors

Several of the consensus statements on concussion reference risk factors such as learning disability, attention-deficit disorder, attention-deficit/ hyperactivity disorder (ADHD), and migraine history (e.g., Giza et al., 2013; P. McCrory et al., 2013, 2017). However, the authors of these statements caution that only limited research supports the role of these factors in modifying concussion recovery or related outcomes. What we do know from our research is that both learning disability and ADHD are associated with worse baseline or preinjury cognitive performance (Elbin et al., 2012). Nelson, Pfaller, Rein, and McCrea (2015) suggested that hyperactivity disorders are related to worse postinjury cognitive impairment, but additional research is needed. Learning disability has received little attention with regard to its effects on postinjury outcomes. However, in an earlier study, we found that football players with learning disability had worse impairment than players without learning disability (M. W. Collins, Grindel, et al., 1999).

Migraine history is another emerging primary risk factor that has limited support in the literature (e.g., Gordon, Dooley, & Wood, 2006). Gordon and colleagues (2006) suggested that a history of migraine was associated with an increase in concussion incidence. Unfortunately, this preliminary finding from a retrospective study has yet to be extended in a prospective study to determine the role of migraine history on concussion-related outcomes. However, the findings from a study of nearly 2,000 pediatric patients with concussion by Heyer, Young, Rose, McNally, and Fischer (2016) suggested that premorbid headaches were unrelated to the development of PTM. This finding is surprising because we recently reported that a familial (personal or immediate family member) history of migraine was associated with a nearly 3 times greater risk of developing PTM following concussion (Sufrinko, McAllister-Deitrick, Elbin, Collins, & Kontos, 2018). Interestingly, we found that familial history of migraine alone was not associated with worse symptoms or impairment. Only when it was associated with PTM did it play an indirect role in worse outcomes following concussion. These findings suggest that the role of migraine in concussion outcomes may be more complicated than previously thought. Clinicians and researchers should consider both personal and family history of migraine as risk factors for poor outcomes following concussion. More research in this area is warranted to better understand the role of migraine and other headache histories on concussion outcomes.

Another factor to consider is history of motion sickness and related vestibular disorders. In our preliminary work in this area, we have reported that patients with a history of motion sickness are nearly 8 times more likely to experience vestibular impairment and symptoms at baseline (Kontos, Sufrinko, Elbin, Puskar, & Collins, 2016). Although this study focused on a preinjury time point, it is reasonable to expect that histories of motion sickness or vestibular disorders also affect postinjury levels of impairment and symptoms in these outcomes. We recently concluded a study that is currently under review, in which we found support for preexisting susceptibility to motion sickness—as reported through a questionnaire—was associated with worse vestibular and oculomotor, but not cognitive, impairment and symptoms following concussion (Sufrinko et al., 2018). This preliminary finding provides further support for primary risk factors driving specific clinical profiles and outcomes in patients following concussion.

Certain preexisting psychological characteristics such as depression (Covassin, Elbin, Larson, & Kontos, 2012) and anxiety (Covassin et al., 2014) have been proposed to influence concussion outcomes. In fact, in our study of depression in more than 1,600 high school and college athletes, we reported that athletes with high depression scores performed worse on visual memory and had more symptoms than those with lower scores (Covassin, Elbin, Larson, & Kontos, 2012). Researchers have also proposed that preexisting sleep disturbances may adversely affect concussion symptoms and related cognitive impairment (Kostyun, 2015). Initial findings from researchers in our clinic support this contention and indicate that the number of sleep-related symptoms and the duration of sleep in combination may be useful in predicting cognitive impairment (Sufrinko, Johnson, & Henry, 2016). There is growing empirical evidence for the above risk factors, which should be considered in patients with concussion.

Researchers have long suggested that genetics plays a role in concussion and related outcomes (e.g., Jordan et al., 1997). Among the genetic factors for which empirical studies offer support are apolipoprotein (*ApoE*) *e4* allele and *ApoE* promoter (*G-219T* polymorphism; Terrell et al., 2008; Tierney et al., 2010) and Tau (Terrell et al., 2008). Preliminary evidence suggests that both the *e4* allele and the *ApoE G-219T* polymorphism are associated with increased risk of concussion (Terrell et al., 2008; Tierney et al., 2010). However, some researchers have reported contrary findings for both the *e4* allele (Kristman et al., 2008) and Tau (Kristman et al., 2008; Terrell et al., 2008), and these studies are limited because of small sample sizes. Larger scale research that examines the interaction of genetics and environmental and other injury characteristics is needed to better develop phenotypes (the observable manifestation in patients) of this injury. Finally, other genetics-related factors, including insulinlike growth factor-1 (IGF-1), IGF binding protein-2, fibroblast growth factor, Cu-Zn superoxide dismutase, superoxide dismutase-1 (SOD-1), nerve growth factor, glial fibrillary acidic protein (GFAP) and S-100, also merit attention from researchers. Regardless, the role of genetic factors such as *ApoE* and Tau in concussion remains unclear.

Emerging Secondary Risk Factors

With regard to secondary risk factors, the initial presentation of a concussion may provide an indication of prognosis. Specifically, the presence of certain signs immediately following an injury, such as posttraumatic amnesia (Chrisman, Rivara, Schiff, Zhou, & Comstock, 2013; M. W. Collins et al., 2003), fogginess (Lau, Collins, & Lovell, 2012), or dizziness (Lau, Kontos, Collins, Mucha, & Lovell, 2011), may be a portent of poor outcomes. However, other factors previously thought to be associated with poor outcomes following concussion (e.g., brief LOC) may be unrelated. In fact, some immediate signs of concussion (e.g., brief LOC, vomiting), which are overt, may result in more conservative initial management and do not seem to be related to worse outcomes as previously reported (e.g., Erlanger, Kaushik, et al., 2003). In fact, we found that both of these signs were protective (i.e., associated with a lower risk) factors for recovery time (Lau, Kontos, et al., 2011). In the case of brief LOC, the temporary shutting down of the brain may also negate some of the initial metabolic effects of the injury. More research is needed to better understand the effects brief LOC and other overt signs and symptoms have on the management of patients with concussion as well as the underlying effects on the injury process in the brain.

Other secondary risk factors include symptom burden or amount and severity of initial symptoms (Casson, Sethi, & Meehan, 2015; McCrea et al., 2013; Meehan, Mannix, Stracciolini, Elbin, & Collins, 2013; Merritt & Arnett, 2014). Patients who have substantial initial symptoms might be managed more conservatively than patients with minimal symptoms. In addition, a high symptom burden, particularly somatic symptoms, may reflect a more severe injury (Howell, O'Brien, Beasley, Mannix, & Meehan, 2016; Iverson, Gardner, McCrory, Zafonte, & Castellani, 2015).

It is certainly possible that some patients may be reporting high levels of symptoms because they are somaticizers, and they might report high levels of symptoms all of the time, but particularly at times of injury or illness (Root et al., 2016). Consequently, a brief assessment of general symptoms may be warranted to determine whether the symptom burden is injury related (see Chapter 4, this volume). The concept of being asymptomatic, therefore, is contingent on preinjury levels of symptoms; not every patient becomes truly asymptomatic following recovery. Instead, these patients are back to normal levels of baseline or preinjury symptoms. Cognitive impairment during the subacute postinjury time period is another factor that has been reported to be associated with prolonged recovery and worse symptoms and impairment (Lau et al., 2012; Lau, Lovell, Collins, & Pardini, 2009).

Some secondary risk factors do not emerge until later in the subacute postinjury time period. One such factor is PTM, which includes headache, nausea, and photosensitivity or phonosensitivity. Researchers have demonstrated that the presence of PTM in the first week following injury is associated with poor outcomes and prolonged recovery (Heyer et al., 2016; Kontos, Elbin, Lau, et al., 2013; Mihalik et al., 2005, 2013). In our study of more than 200 athletes we found that the presence of PTM during this period was predictive of more significant impairment on memory and processing speed, as well as a protracted (> 21 days) recovery time (Kontos, Elbin, Lau, et al., 2013). Individuals with PTM were also worse off than those with non-PTM headache, suggesting that type of headache matters. We also believe that some of the primary risk factors such as sex may be surrogates for other underlying risk factors. For example, females are more likely to have preexisting migraine headache, which may increase the likelihood that they develop PTM. Our recent research suggests that as many as 75% of female patients experience PTM symptom after sustaining a concussion (Snook, Henry, Sanfilippo, Zelznik, & Kontos, 2016). Although additional research is needed, this finding may explain why females experience more pronounced effects from this injury than do males.

Note About Risk Factors in the Recent Concussion in Sport Group Statement

The most recent Concussion in Sport Group (CISG) consensus statement, which came out of the group's fall 2016 meeting in Berlin (P. McCrory et al., 2017), indicates that a high initial symptom burden was a reliable and empirically supported risk factor for poorer outcome and prolonged recovery following concussion. But the consensus statement downplayed the role of other factors such as age, sex, and concussion history. This apparent reduction in support for these risk factors likely reflects an overly strict set of inclusion criteria for studies to be included as evidence, such that only prospective case control studies are being considered by groups like the CISG. However, consensus statements such as that of the CISG also seem to change the rules for other risk factors that have seemingly limited empirical support. For example, and somewhat surprisingly, the 2017 CISG statement states that children, adolescents, and young adults with preexisting mental health or migraine history are at greater risk for prolonged recovery (P. McCrory et al., 2017). However, there is very limited empirical evidence for either of these risk factors. In fact, in our own study of migraine history, we reported that while a history of migraine was associated with increased risk for PTM symptoms, it was not directly associated with prolonged recovery or other adverse outcomes associated with concussion (Sufrinko et al., 2018). This discrepant interpretation of the evidence for risk factors in the extant literature as communicated in the 2017 CISG consensus statement highlights the importance of analyzing the empirical support for each statement independently to verify its accuracy.

CONCUSSION "PLAYS DIRTY"

The effects of concussion often magnify preexisting risk factors or conditions (see Figure 2.7). For example, a patient with a history of migraine may experience exacerbated migraine symptoms following a concussion. Similarly, a patient with a history of motion sickness may experience vestibular deficits and symptoms following the injury. Therefore, we often think of concussion as "playing dirty," by targeting preexisting vulnerabilities, thereby resulting in more significant, though possibly predictable, outcomes following injury. This notion was reinforced in our recent research, in which we examined baseline or preinjury performance on the Vestibular/Ocular Motor Screening (VOMS) tool in relation to preexisting histories of motion sickness and other vestibular disorders (Kontos, Sufrinko, Elbin, et al., 2016). Our findings indicate that individuals with a history of these disorders score at levels commensurate with clinical cutoffs at baseline. This finding, combined with our research on the effects of preexisting PTM and other medical history–related risk factors on VOMS scores (which indicated that these individuals have worse vestibular and oculomotor symptoms and impairment postinjury; Womble et al., 2017), suggest that preexisting issues result in higher levels of impairment in those areas. Regardless of the cause, awareness of preexisting issues can provide insight into subsequent impairment, symptoms, and prognosis for recovery time.

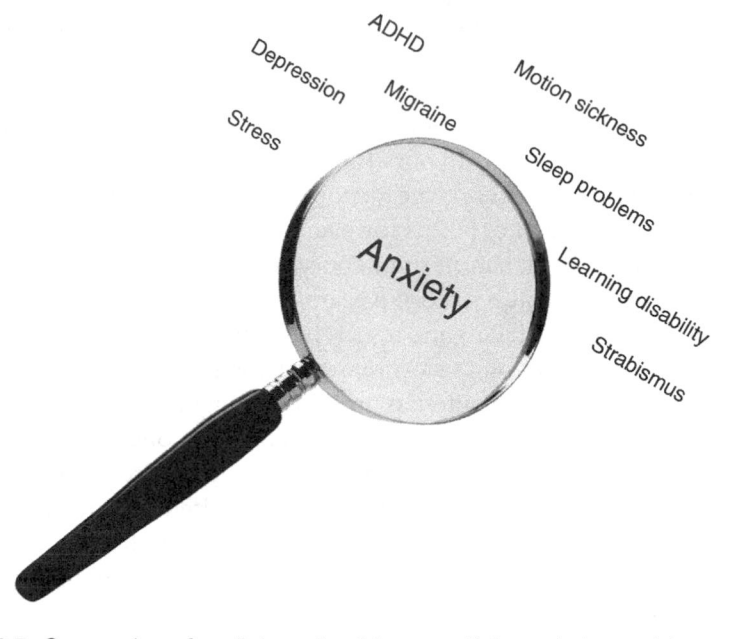

Figure 2.7. Concussion often "plays dirty" by magnifying existing problems. ADHD = attention-deficit/hyperactivity disorder.

Recovery Time After a Concussion

Recovery time following a concussion varies according to the nature of the injury, primary (e.g., age, sex, concussion history) and secondary (e.g., symptom burden, dizziness, PTM symptoms, continuing to play the sport) risk factors, initial identification and clinical care, and other factors. Historically, concussion recovery was considered to take on average 7 to 10 days (P. McCrory et al., 2013). However, our view has shifted to suggest that recovery takes longer (see Henry et al., 2016). In fact, in the recent CISG consensus documents, recovery for adults was estimated to be 14 days on average (P. McCrory et al., 2017), whereas for children and adolescents it was estimated to be 4 weeks (Davis et al., 2017). These changes in perceptions of average recovery time following concussion reflect our growing understanding that recovery is individualized based on risk factors.

Long-Term Effects of Concussion

Long term effects of concussion can be divided into two categories: prolonged postinjury sequelae and chronic or residual effects. The former are best characterized by the term *postconcussion symptoms* (PCS), previously referred to as *postconcussion syndrome*. In short, many patients (about 20%–30%) experience lingering deficits and symptoms following a concussion (P. McCrory et al., 2013). If not properly identified and treated with targeted approaches, these sequelae may last months to over a year in some cases. We have seen many patients in our clinic who have been mismanaged with repeated prescriptions of rest over a course of several months, resulting in unnecessary development of PCS. However, some patients simply take longer to recover because of risk factors or phenotypes such as migraine history, age, gender, and motion sickness history. Regardless of the etiology of PCS, it warrants attention from clinicians and researchers. In contrast, potential chronic or residual effects from concussion represent long-term neurodegenerative changes to the brain that manifest as progressive impairments and symptoms. Chronic traumatic encephalopathy (CTE) represents one extreme example of these chronic effects that have been proposed by researchers to be related to concussion. Although evidence for CTE is limited and misinformation abounds, it represents a significant issue that warrants further discussion. However, we will first discuss the more immediate and treatable prolonged effects of concussion known as PCS.

Postconcussion Symptoms

The presence of PCS is based on a variety of lingering symptoms and deficits, including headache, sleep disturbance, mood changes, difficulty concentrating, and fatigue (Leddy, Sandhu, Sodhi, Baker, & Willer, 2012). On the surface, PCS can mimic other diagnoses, including chronic pain disorder, anxiety, depression, and somatization disorders. As such, it is important for clinicians to first determine using a thorough interview and assessment whether a patient is experiencing PCS or some other issue. There is some debate as to when one can accurately refer to PCS; some researchers have argued that PCS only applies to patients after a time period of 3 or more months following a concussion (Binder, Rohling, & Larrabee, 1997). More recent clinical approaches focus on prolonged recovery times beyond a normal recovery trajectory, which may vary from 10 to 30 days depending on risk factors and the domain being measured to determine recovery (Henry, Burkhart, Elbin, Agarwal, & Kontos, 2015). The nature of the concussion and typical recovery time (e.g., motor vehicle collision with longer or shorter recovery times) may also influence this time frame for a determination of PCS. In any case, PCS is a problem for many patients following concussion. In our experience, one of the universal themes for patients with PCS is a self-imposed or in some cases prescribed reduction in normal activities (both physical and cognitive) that seems to feed or exacerbate their PCS. Patients with PCS are often fatigued, have poor sleep patterns, and lack the energy to engage in normal activities. The resulting lack of activity further feeds the cycle of PCS by providing fewer distractions from and more time to ruminate on the symptoms. In addition, the lack of activity furthers physical deconditioning for patients, thereby resulting in a vicious cycle (see Figure 2.8). As such, the conundrum for clinicians is to get patients with PCS active at a time when they lack the energy to be active on their own. The good news is that prescribed active approaches to treatment can accelerate recovery in these patients. Specifically, vestibular, ocular/vision, and psychoeducational treatments may improve recovery in patients with PCS (Leddy, Baker, & Willer, 2016). Prescribed exercise, which may improve cerebrovascular blood flow, has been shown to improve symptoms in patients with PCS (Baker, Freitas, Leddy, Kozlowski, & Willer, 2012). However, these active approaches fly in the face of conventional wisdom for prescribed rest for the "miserable minority" of patients with PCS. Consequently, additional research to substantiate and refine the use of prescribed activity for patients with PCS is warranted.

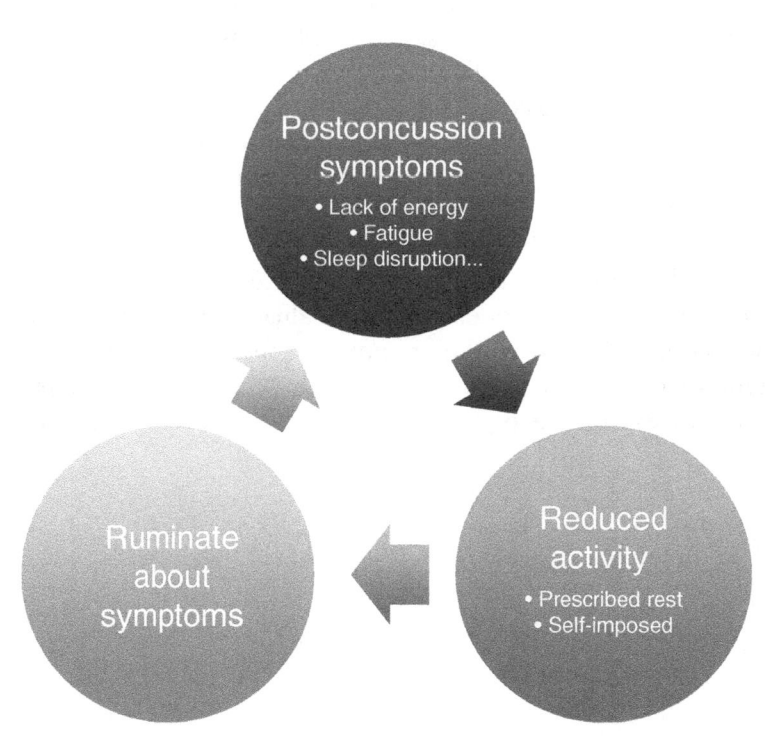

Figure 2.8. Vicious cycle of postconcussion symptoms.

CONCLUSION

Current concussion definitions are constantly evolving. The most elegant among them bear a remarkable similarity to their historical predecessors. Concussions involve linear and rotational mechanical forces that cause axonal tearing/shearing and contusions in the brain. These forces result in neurometabolic, cytotoxic, and cerebrovascular effects; and subtle damage to white matter in the brain. Concussion is characterized by an energy crisis in the brain, wherein energy demand outstrips energy supply.

However, despite similar underlying mechanisms, patients with concussion present with individualized and myriad symptoms. These patients initially present with a global constellation of symptoms, with subsequent more distinct symptom clusters. The time since injury plays a role in symptoms, and certain individual symptoms (e.g., dizziness) and clusters of symptoms (e.g., PTM) may be more important at various postinjury time points than others. Both established and emerging risk factors are critical to understanding a patient's clinical trajectory following concussion. Adolescents, females, and individuals with a history of concussion (particularly mismanaged concussions) seem to be more at risk from the effects of this injury. Emerging risk factors such as dizziness, fogginess, and PTM are associated with prolonged recovery and poor outcome following injury.

Prognosis following concussion is based in part on a patient's risk profile (or what they bring to the table). Although most concussions resolve within a month, PCS affect a large number of patients and warrants attention from clinicians and researchers. As we continue to learn more about recovery time and risk profiles, we will be able to better manage expectations about recovery and develop more effective and earlier treatments for patients with this injury. However, to better understand and evaluate risk factors and the effects of concussion, and to develop more precise approaches to its treatment, a comprehensive, interdisciplinary assessment is warranted (see Chapter 4). In Chapter 3, we explore the psychological issues associated with concussion.

3

PSYCHOLOGICAL ISSUES ASSOCIATED WITH CONCUSSION

Psychological symptoms are common after concussion. In fact, our research suggests that 29% of patients experience one or more psychological symptoms (e.g., sadness, more emotional, nervous, irritable) following their injury (see Table 2.2; Kontos, Elbin, et al., 2012). Among the more common psychological issues following concussion are mood-related changes, including depression (e.g., Kontos, Covassin, Elbin, & Parker, 2012), anxiety (e.g., Iverson & Lange, 2003), and posttraumatic stress (e.g., Kontos, Kotwal, et al., 2013). From a clinical profile perspective, the anxiety/mood profile for patients sustaining concussion includes anxiety and depression. Patients often present with an anxiety/mood clinical profile concurrently with other clinical profiles. However, the anxiety/mood profile and other concomitant psychological issues may be the primary or only profile present. In many of these cases, clinicians must determine whether the patient is experiencing these psychological issues as a result of the concussion, whether these issues

http://dx.doi.org/10.1037/0000087-004

Concussion: A Clinical Profile Approach to Assessment and Treatment, by A. P. Kontos and M. W. Collins

were present prior to their concussion, or whether they may have developed after the concussion but independently from it.

DISENTANGLING PSYCHOLOGICAL AND CONCUSSION SYMPTOMS

One of the biggest challenges to clinicians working with patients following concussion is disentangling concussion symptoms from psychological issues. Many concussion symptoms, such as fatigue and dizziness, are common in psychological disorders, including depression, anxiety, and posttraumatic stress. In addition, sleep problems (e.g., more or less sleep, poor sleep quality) are common for patients with concussion as well as psychological disorders (see Figure 3.1). In addition to symptoms, many of the impairments that are common with concussion (including deficits in memory, attention, executive function, and balance) often overlap with psychological disorders. This overlap in symptoms and impairment highlights the need for a comprehensive assessment; we discuss this in Chapter 4. The approach to assessment should control for other symptoms or impairment that are either preexisting or related to other conditions.

In summary, we need to be able to boil symptoms and impairments down to those that are specific to the concussive injury. The key to determining the etiology of psychological issues in patients following concussion is to establish a chronological history of psychological issues specific to each patient. A good place to start this process is to examine personality traits.

PERSONALITY AND CONCUSSION

Each patient has unique personality traits that can interact with the concussion to influence symptoms, impairment, clinical profiles, and the effectiveness of therapies and other interventions. For example, a patient who is trait anxious is likely to present with elevated anxiety following a concussion. Again, concussion plays dirty and often magnifies preexisting vulnerabilities or characteristics, whether they are physiological, such as vestibular disorders, or psychological, such as anxiety.

Unfortunately, there is limited research on personality and concussion outcomes. In a study of healthy collegiate athletes, Merritt, Rabinowitz, and Arnett (2015) reported that the Neuroticism and Agreeableness personality factors on the NEO Five Factor Inventory (McCrae & Costa, 2004) were predictive of higher symptoms scores on the Post-Concussion Symptom Scale (Lovell et al., 2006). Clarke, Genat, and Anderson (2012) reported similar

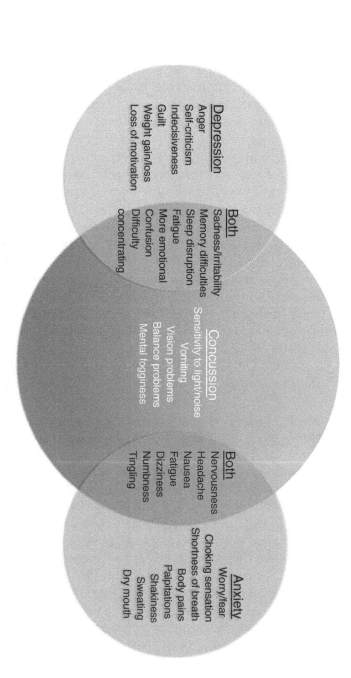

Figure 3.1. Overlap among symptoms of concussion, anxiety, and depression.

Depression
Anger
Self-criticism
Indecisiveness
Guilt
Weight gain/loss
Loss of motivation

Both
Sadness/irritability
Memory difficulties
Sleep disruption
Fatigue
More emotional
Confusion
Difficulty
concentrating

Concussion
Sensitivity to light/noise
Vomiting
Vision problems
Balance problems
Mental fogginess

Both
Nervousness
Headache
Nausea
Fatigue
Dizziness
Numbness
Tingling

Anxiety
Worry/fear
Choking sensation
Shortness of breath
Body pains
Palpitations
Shakiness
Sweating
Dry mouth

findings for neuroticism in a study comparing adult patients with mild traumatic brain injury (TBI), spinal injury, and controls. However, they combined anxiety and depression with neuroticism because of the small sample size ($N = 60$ divided into three groups), so it is unclear which factors influenced their findings. Given the relationship between baseline symptom scores and postconcussion symptoms and impairment we reported in our research (Custer et al., 2016; see also Chapter 4, this volume), it is intuitive to infer that these same personality factors would influence postconcussion outcomes too.

Researchers have also examined the relationship of *anxiety sensitivity*, which refers to an individual's fear associated with bodily sensations, and *alexithymia*, or one's inability to identify physical feelings and emotional arousal to postconcussion outcomes (Wood, O'Hagan, Williams, McCabe, & Chadwick, 2014). In their study, Wood and colleagues (2014) compared patients with controls and reported that both higher anxiety sensitivity and alexithymia were associated with higher anxiety sensitivity, alexithymia, psychological distress, and postconcussion symptoms in the concussion group than controls. Also within the concussion group, higher scores on both factors were associated with higher symptoms and psychological distress following their injury.

Other researchers have reported contrary findings for some personality characteristics. For example, in a study looking at explanatory style, or optimism versus pessimism, Shapcott, Bloom, Johnston, Loughead, and Delaney (2007) reported that more optimistic style was associated with longer recovery and higher symptoms but not increased risk for concussion. These researchers speculated that because concussion involves more frustrating and unclear recovery, patients who are usually optimistic may become frustrated and experience psychological distress following a concussion, thereby prolonging their recovery. Although this explanation makes sense, it is likely that some personality factors may not influence concussion outcomes, even psychological issues.

Another personality trait, somatization, has recently begun to receive attention from researchers (e.g., Grubenhoff et al., 2016; Root et al., 2016). Somatization is characterized by a tendency to internalize problems and manifest them as physical complaints and symptoms. In both our study (Root et al., 2016) and a similar study by Grubenhoff and colleagues (2016), pediatric patients with high somatization scores on the Children's Somatization Inventory (L. S. Walker & Garber, 2003) took longer to recover and reported higher symptoms following a concussion. In the Grubenhoff et al. study nearly 33% of patients were still symptomatic at 1 month. Interestingly, state anxiety also influenced prolonged symptoms in this study, suggesting that somaticizers may also be more likely to present with mood/anxiety clinical profiles following concussion. Clearly, more research in this area is needed. In any case, clinicians should consider the role of personality traits and other patient psychological tendencies on concussion outcomes. Use of somatization measures such as the Children's Somatization Inventory and the somatization subscale of the Brief Symptom Inventory-18 (Derogatis, 2001) is also advised (see Chapter 4).

PSYCHOLOGICAL RESPONSES TO CONCUSSION

Several models of psychological antecedents and responses to injury have been proposed in the sport psychology literature (see Wiese-Bjornstal, Smith, Shaffer, & Morrey, 1998, and J. Williams & Andersen, 1998, for thorough reviews). However, these models have yet to be applied to patients with concussion, which is somewhat surprising because their theoretical underpinning might provide a better understanding of the mechanisms and potential interventions for the psychological issues that often accompany concussion. For example, J. Williams and Andersen's (1998) stress model of injury may help to explain such concussion risk factors as personality (e.g., anxiety), history of stressors (e.g., daily hassles), and coping resources (e.g., low social support). In addition, this model provides a framework for understanding the role of the interaction between an individual's cognitive appraisal (e.g., worry about being injured) and their physiological (e.g., overarousal) and attentional changes (e.g., narrow focus of attention) that might lead to injury.

Although the stress model was intended to predict psychological risk for an injury occurring in sport, we believe it is equally applicable to nonsport populations and in predicting a poor response to an injury such as a concussion after it has occurred. In this regard, the model can be viewed as a framework for understanding the factors that might influence secondary risk for poor outcomes, particularly those that are psychological in nature. For example, a patient who is anxious, who has limited social support, and who is convinced that the injury is going to cause long-term neurological damage may struggle following a concussion. Add worry about returning to work or school and concomitant higher levels of stress to these underlying issues, and you have a recipe for a poor outcome following concussion. Specifically, this patient may respond with increased anxiety, mood, and other psychological responses related to their concussion that can hinder recovery, reduce adherence to rehabilitation and therapies, and delay return to normal activity.

With regard to the psychological response to injury, in their integrated model of response to injury in sport, Wiese-Bjornstal and colleagues (1998) posited that a variety of factors could influence an injured athlete's responses. As with the previously described stress model, we believe that the integrated model can also be applied to concussion in nonsport populations. The integrated model suggests that after an injury, or a concussion in this case, an individual's responses are dictated by personal (e.g., demographic, psychological) and situational (e.g., social, environment) factors that interact to influence their cognitive appraisal (e.g., perceived length of recovery, perceived control or attribution for rehabilitation and recovery) of their concussion. These factors combine with the patient's behavioral (e.g., adherence, malingering, risk taking) and emotional (e.g., fear of reinjury, frustration with slow recovery process) responses to determine physical and psychological recovery outcomes. Both the stress and integrated models require greater attention from concussion researchers and clinicians and should be applied to the design of studies to better understand the psychological antecedents and responses to concussion. One factor not considered in the preceding models, but that we believe plays a significant role in the response to and recovery from a concussion, is sleep.

Sleep Overlay

As discussed in Chapter 1, sleep problems are common following concussion and may occur concurrently with any of the concussion clinical profiles described previously. In fact, it is estimated that between 30% and 80% of patients experience sleep problems following concussion or mild TBI (Tkachenko, Singh, Hasanaj, Serrano, & Kothare, 2016). Although sleep problems may not constitute a psychological issue per se, they may exacerbate a patient's psychological issues following a concussion, much as they do for symptoms and cognitive impairment (Sufrinko, Pearce, et al., 2015). For other patients, sleep problems may be a result of psychological issues such as depression or anxiety. Irrespective of the source, quality of sleep is compromised in many patients following concussion. In some cases, these sleep problems may manifest as a sleep disorder.

Among the sleep disorders that patients may experience following concussion are hypersomnia, insomnia, parasomnias, and sleep apnea (Wickwire et al., 2016). Patients may also experience circadian disruption to their sleep–wakefulness cycles. In our experience, this effect seems to be exacerbated by frequent napping. Researchers have indicated that certain injury-related and other factors may increase the likelihood of sleep disorders following a concussion. In a retrospective study of 93 patients seen at the emergency department, researchers reported that having moderate to severe headache, dizziness, or psychiatric symptoms was associated with increased risk for sleep problems following concussion (Tkachenko et al., 2016). In addition, motor vehicle accidents and medications prescribed in the emergency department were positively related to sleep problems. These findings suggest that both the mechanism of injury and the initial pharmacological treatment may contribute to sleep problems in patients following concussion.

It would seem logical that preexisting sleep problems would worsen post-concussion sleep problems. Our research seems to bear this out with patients who report preinjury sleep problems experiencing worse symptoms and cognitive impairment within the first week of sustaining a concussion (Sufrinko, Pearce et al., 2015) Surprisingly, however, acute sleep deprivation in animal model research seems to have the paradoxical effect of protecting rats from more severe brain injury (Moldovan et al., 2010). It is thought that this effect may be the result of a preconditioning to the potential ischemic effects of brain injury. Initial clinical research of more than 500 adolescents with a concussion suggested that sleeping less than 7 hours the night after their injury was associated with higher symptom reporting following their injury but no other adverse outcomes (Kostyun, Milewski, & Hafeez, 2015). However, the researchers also reported that sleeping more than 9 hours the night after sustaining a concussion was associated with worse cognitive impairment following their injury (Kostyun et al., 2015). As such, additional research in this area in patients is warranted before clinicians start depriving patients of sleep to reduce the effects of concussion.

Typically, sleep has been viewed as a symptom of concussion, but some researchers have suggested that sleep should instead be conceptualized as a modifiable factor that can be treated, thereby accelerating recovery from concussion (Wickwire et al., 2016). Sleep problems following concussion may also directly influence psychological issues and be challenging to treat, especially for patients experiencing depression or posttraumatic stress or for those with concomitant physical injuries, such as a fractured femur resulting from a motor vehicle accident (Wickwire et al., 2016). In conclusion, clinicians and researchers alike need to better understand the role of preexisting and postconcussion sleep problems to assess and treat psychological issues following this injury.

Depression

Changes in mood are among the most common psychological sequelae reported by patients following a concussion. Researchers have documented changes in mood (Mainwaring et al., 2004) and depression (Kontos, Covassin, Elbin, & Parker, 2012) immediately following concussion. It is estimated that approximately 6% of patients with concussion experience clinical levels of depression following their injury (Jorge & Robinson, 2002). These numbers underscore the clinical relevance of understanding changes in mood in patients following a concussion.

Depression following a concussion may result from a number of causes. Patients may experience transient changes in areas of the brain associated with depression including the amygdala, hippocampus, and dorsolateral prefrontal cortex (J. K. Chen, Johnston, Petrides, & Ptito, 2008; Sheline, Wang,

Gado, Csernansky, & Vannier, 1996). Depression may also be the result of a psychological response to injury related to the injury response, withdrawal from sport, or frustration associated with an often uncertain and ambiguous recovery process (Kontos, Covassin, et al., 2012). In addition, we believe that the inactive approaches (i.e., cognitive and physical rest) usually prescribed following a concussion may be especially detrimental to patients who are experiencing an anxiety/mood concussion clinical profile. The additional time to ruminate about symptoms, functional impairment with no concomitant visible injury, and perception that there is nothing they can do to get better may all contribute to patients' feelings of depression following a concussion. As mentioned earlier, discriminating depression from other concussion-related symptoms is challenging given the overlap of symptoms common to both, such as changes in mood, confusion, and drowsiness/fatigue.

A history of depression makes the process of discerning the symptoms resulting from concussion compared to those from mood disorder or related issues more challenging for the clinician and highlights the importance of a thorough clinical interview and exam, including a detailed psychosocial history. Depression following a concussion may originate from a preexisting mood disorder or dysthymic predisposition. In fact, our study of baseline depression levels in more than 1,600 collegiate and high school athletes (Kontos, Covassin, et al., 2012) revealed that 2% of the total sample reported moderate to severe depression, and those with severe depression scores (> 29 on the Beck Depression Inventory–II [BDI-II]; Beck, Steer, & Brown, 1996) scored worse on cognitive tests like visual memory. Moreover, women reported higher levels than did men, and adolescents were higher than college-aged athletes.

Research on depression following concussion is limited. We prospectively examined depression using the BDI-II following concussion in a multisite study of adolescent and collegiate athletes (Kontos, Covassin, et al., 2012). Depression symptoms on the BDI-II rose after concussion and persisted up to 14 days postinjury. However, the levels of depression, though higher than baseline, were in most instances well below clinical levels, with most averaging minimal to mild. We found that only three patients reported postconcussion levels of depression (i.e., moderate on BDI-II) that warranted a follow-up mental health referral. Surprisingly, females in our study reported the same levels of depression as males. Also of note, we found that college-aged patients continued to experience an elevation in symptoms at 14 days, whereas adolescents had returned to baseline levels by the same time. This finding suggests a potential growing frustration with their injury and recovery in college-aged athletes.

Other researchers have reported generally similar findings for depression and mood following concussion. For example, Mainwaring and colleagues (2004) found that college athletes reported mood disturbance including depression symptoms and confusion up to 3 weeks from injury. However, this study did not report clinical levels of depression. Also, in a follow-up study, Mainwaring, Hutchison, Bisschop, Comper, and Richards (2010) reported that changes in depression and mood following a concussion resolved on average quicker than did cognitive impairment (7–14 days vs. 25 days). Missing from these studies are long-term follow-ups to determine whether depressive and other mood symptoms lingered. In one study of more than 300 active duty military personnel, researchers reported that depressive symptoms and posttraumatic stress disorder (PTSD) improved only marginally within 5 years of the concussion (MacDonald et al., 2014). The researchers suggested that earlier identification and treatment of psychological issues such as depression are warranted and may reduce the effects they reported. Similarly, in a more recent study of nearly 700 youth ice hockey players, those with a history of concussion were more likely to report psychological sequelae, including depression (Mrazik, Brooks, Jubinville, Meeuwisse, & Emery, 2016). In light of these findings, additional research on residual mood changes and depression is needed.

Anxiety and Posttraumatic Stress

Anxiety is a common psychological issue following concussion and comprises the anxiety/mood clinical profiles described in Chapter 1. It is also a profile that may occur with other cognitive difficulties (Iverson, 2006). Proposed mechanisms for anxiety after a concussion include the cognitive appraisal of the concussion that results in worry, low perceived control, fatigue, and apprehension about the injury and recovery. A patient may also have anxiety because of the physiological consequences from the brain injury. For example, symptoms that can be both debilitating and uncontrollable, such as headache, dizziness, or vertigo, may provoke anxiety in patients that can quickly generalize beyond the injury and its effects. Similar to anxiety, posttraumatic stress symptoms and PTSD (the diagnosed disorder) may manifest in patients who sustain concussion. Concussions that involve significant trauma, such as those resulting from motor vehicle collisions, blast explosions, and assaults, may be more likely to cause posttraumatic stress symptoms. Whereas considerable attention has been paid to posttraumatic stress and mild TBI since the wars in Afghanistan and Iraq, little attention has been paid to anxiety and concussion.

Researchers have only recently begun to focus on anxiety and concussion. Earlier studies by Iverson and Lange (2003) and Kashluba and colleagues (2004) suggested that anxiety did indeed occur in patients following a concussion. Grubenhoff et al. (2016) reported that among 179 children with a concussion, higher state anxiety scores were associated with delayed (i.e., still symptomatic at 1-month postinjury) symptom resolution. Other researchers have identified a relevant set of risk factors to consider when evaluating the risk of anxiety in patients with concussion, including being female, a higher initial postconcussion symptom score, a higher emotional postconcussion symptom score, and a personal or familial history of a psychological disorder (Ellis, Ritchie, et al., 2015). The latter factors (personal or familial history of psychological disorder) should be included in any medical and psychosocial history. Although this study focused on children, it is likely that these same risk factors would also be relevant in adult populations.

Some researchers have begun to suggest a link between anxiety and depression following concussion. In a study of baseline and postconcussion anxiety and depression in 67 collegiate athletes, J. Yang, Peek-Asa, Covassin, and Torner (2015) found that depression scores and anxiety scores were positively correlated with each other following a concussion. They also reported that baseline depression was the best predictor of postconcussion depression and anxiety, suggesting that depression and anxiety should be viewed in concert rather than independently in patients who sustained concussion. Not all research on anxiety and concussion has demonstrated a link. In fact, in a large study of 341 adults aged 17 and older from New Zealand, the researchers reported that residual levels of anxiety at 1-year postconcussion were not different from the general population (Theadom et al., 2016).

The majority of research on concussion and posttraumatic stress or its clinical cousin PTSD has involved military personnel. Recent research using structured clinical interviews indicated that slightly more than 60% of 107 active duty military personnel and veterans were diagnosed with at least one anxiety or mood disorder related episode during a 2-year period (W. C. Walker, Franke, McDonald, Sima, & Keyser-Marcus, 2015). Surprisingly, this study did not report a link between blast mild TBI (i.e., mild TBI that is directly or indirectly caused by exposure to blast force from an explosion) or mild TBI and these diagnoses, suggesting that other mechanisms for these psychological disorders may be involved. We reported similar results from our prospective research of 136 U.S. Army Special Operations Forces personnel in that previous exposure to blast mild TBI was unrelated to PTSD following subsequent mild TBI (Manners et al., 2016). However, we found that pre-injury posttraumatic stress and concussion symptoms, and positive radiologic findings accurately identified PTSD following concussion (Manners et al., 2016). This population is selected for high resiliency, and so it is noteworthy that 11% of personnel met criteria for posttraumatic stress symptoms even before injury.

We have observed that some patients with vestibular clinical profiles experience anxiety (Kontos, McAllister-Deitrick, & Reynolds, 2016). For some patients, this concurrent anxiety may be a direct consequence of a central vestibular impairment following their injury. For other patients, it may result from a perceived loss of control or from fear associated with the unpredictable nature of periodic vertigo or dizziness symptoms. This anxiety may then extend to environments or triggers associated with the onset of vestibular symptoms. For example, driving a car may elicit anxiety as a result of the anticipated symptoms of dizziness associated with this activity. In these cases, it is critical to treat the underlying vestibular impairment and symptoms first, to determine the source of the anxiety. If the anxiety persists, then additional treatment is warranted.

Conversion Disorder

Most patients who experience postconcussion psychological issues present with either mood (e.g., depression) or anxiety-based problems. A less common occurrence is conversion disorder, which involves presentation of symptoms, sensory disturbance, or movement impairment not attributable to an underlying neurological cause or malingering, but attributed to psychological causes. Trauma and injuries such as concussion are often a trigger for a conversion disorder (Hallett et al., 2006). A search of the literature revealed only one published case study of a visual conversion disorder secondary to a concussion following a motor vehicle accident (Foutch, 2015). This reported case, which involved symptoms of unilateral blindness in the right eye with equivocal support for neurological and organic causes, was not only fascinating to read but revealed the potential for conversion disorder following concussion. In this case, the patient, an adult woman, was dealing with multiple psychological stressors including the recent death of her father, current deployment of her husband, isolation with her infant child, and the motor vehicle accident that resulted in a concussion. The manifestation of these psychological stressors resulted in the visual conversion disorder, which resolved immediately after the patient discussed her stressors with her optometrist.

Additional published case studies and empirical research on the prevalence and etiology of conversion disorder in patients with concussion are needed. Until then, clinicians should be aware of this rare psychological issue that may accompany concussion, particularly when other psychological issues may be present as in the case described above.

Malingering

Confirmed malingering related to physical or mental disability results in up to $55.5 billion in direct and indirect costs to society in the United States each year (Chafetz, 2011). Although the exact cost from malingering attributable to concussion is unknown, it is likely a growing concern for insurance companies because, much like a lower back or cervical injury, concussion diagnosis and recovery can be challenging to confirm or refute. Malingering involves fabricated or exaggerated physical or psychological symptoms and impairment for some external gain, including but not limited to financial gain (e.g., worker's compensation, disability claim), escape (e.g., getting out of military duty), and attention from others (e.g., from physicians, family, athletic trainers). Another common indicator of malingering is poor effort on tests. As a result, effort-based testing to detect malingering was developed, including the Test of Memory Malingering (Tombaugh, 1997) and the Dot Counting Test (Boone et al., 2002). Ideally tests of effort or malingering should be quick and involve automatic performances or responses (Silver, 2012).

Malingering following a concussion may range from extending one's recovery by exaggerating symptoms to completely fabricating an injury and its effects when no organic injury actually occurred. Certain factors such as pending litigation and compensation and injury may increase the likelihood of malingering. Researchers have shown that litigation is associated with higher levels of symptoms, particularly anxiety, and worse concussion outcomes (Feinstein, Ouchterlony, Somerville, & Jardine, 2001). In our experience, the mechanism of injury may play a role in malingering, with concussion from motor vehicle collision, falls, and assaults being more likely to result in malingering than sport-related injuries. In fact, if anything, athletes may do the opposite and minimize their symptoms and try to cover up impairment so they can return sooner to sport. Apparent malingering may be associated with the stereotype threat, wherein a patient thinks that because of his concussion he should be symptomatic and impaired and therefore almost subconsciously behaves accordingly (Silver, 2012). Malingering may provide secondary gain, such as attention from medical staff or an escape from sport or military duty. After all, it is easier to save face through malingering than to admit disinterest in or displeasure with a chosen activity. Consequently, clinicians should consider multiple reasons for poor performance or symptoms following a concussion before settling on malingering as the cause.

Suicide

The relationship between suicide and concussion is not well understood. However, suicide is strongly related to psychological disorders and therefore warrants attention from clinicians working with patients following a concussion who are experiencing psychological issues. Researchers have reported an association between mild TBI and suicide in military populations (e.g., Hoge et al., 2008). However, in this population it is often difficult to extricate whether the suicide is related to mild TBI, posttraumatic stress, or some other comorbid condition.

Researchers have begun to examine the association between concussion and suicide in civilian populations. In an epidemiological study of patients with concussion in Ontario, Fralick, Thiruchelvam, Tien, and Redelmeier (2016) reported that suicide rates over a 9-year follow-up period were 3 times higher for patients who had a concussion than population norms. Patients with depression have an increased risk of attempting suicide, and given that some patients experience depression and other mood changes following a concussion, as discussed earlier in this chapter, an evaluation of suicide in these patients is particularly indicated. As Fralick et al. (2016) reported, being male and having a history of a psychological disorder were additional risk factors for suicide following a concussion, further supporting the comprehensive assessment described in Chapter 4 of this volume. Fralick et al. also reported that concussions occurring on the weekend resulted in a 33% increase in risk of suicide compared with those occurring on weekdays. When considering suicide and concussion, it is important to note that the effects reported in Fralick et al. represent one study, are not causal, and may have been confounded by other suicide risk factors. Moreover, the risk was spread over a 9-year period, during which many events that contributed to suicide risk could have transpired. Nevertheless, suicide is a rare but possible consequence for patients following concussion that warrants attention from clinicians and researchers.

CONCLUSION

Many patients experience psychological symptoms and issues following concussion that often overlap with other concussion symptoms. When attempting to disentangle psychological symptoms, it is important to consider the interaction between the person and the injury itself. In addition, patients may have different psychological responses to their concussion. As such, theories from sport psychology that focus on psychological response to injury may be useful in better understanding the antecedents and outcomes related to different responses. Sleep disruption following concussion is nearly ubiquitous and should always be evaluated and treated to facilitate recovery. Depression, anxiety, and posttraumatic stress can complicate recovery following concussion and should not be overlooked in patients with this injury. In more extreme cases, patients may develop conversion disorder following a concussion. More commonly, patients may engage in malingering, particularly when there is secondary gain associated with this behavior. Although rare, risk of suicide following concussion should be monitored and emergent care provided when warranted.

4

COMPREHENSIVE ASSESSMENT OF CONCUSSION

Many areas of medicine and research have *gold standards*, measures with which all other similar measures are compared for validity. For example, the gold standard to assess body composition is hydrostatic (underwater) displacement. However, this process is expensive, time-consuming, and daunting: Subjects have to hold their breath under water and then expel all of their air while remaining under water. It sounds easy enough, but the underwater test produces high anxiety in many people. Consequently, researchers developed skin calipers to measure body composition that are simpler, less time-consuming, and less daunting. Assessing concussion effects in the brain is more complicated than determining body composition, and we do not yet have a gold standard for assessing concussion.

Some researchers have argued that the current standard for concussion revolves around symptom assessments (Randolph et al., 2009). However, as we discussed previously, self-reported symptoms do not always provide the most accurate and reliable source of information regarding a concussion and

http://dx.doi.org/10.1037/0000087-005
Concussion: A Clinical Profile Approach to Assessment and Treatment, by A. P. Kontos and M. W. Collins

its effects (Elbin, Knox, et al., 2016). In lieu of a gold standard, clinicians have typically relied on symptom reports as well as cognitive and balance performance to assess concussion (P. McCrory et al., 2013). Consequently, researchers and entrepreneurs have developed and marketed a variety of "concussion tests" that run the gamut of simple reaction time tasks to elaborate blood biomarker tests. As a result, there is a persistent misconception among the public and media that a "silver bullet" concussion assessment exists right around the corner. However, given the different clinical profiles following concussion (see Chapter 1), it is unlikely that a single approach to assessing this injury can be effective for all patients. Therefore, a comprehensive approach to assessing concussion is warranted.

A comprehensive approach to assessing concussion is intuitive and flows from the clinical profiles discussed in the preceding chapter. Concussion assessments should cover a variety of domains that are affected following a concussion. Those domains include (a) symptoms, (b) cognitive, (c) neuromotor, (d) vestibular/oculomotor (vision), and (e) psychological (see Figure 4.1).

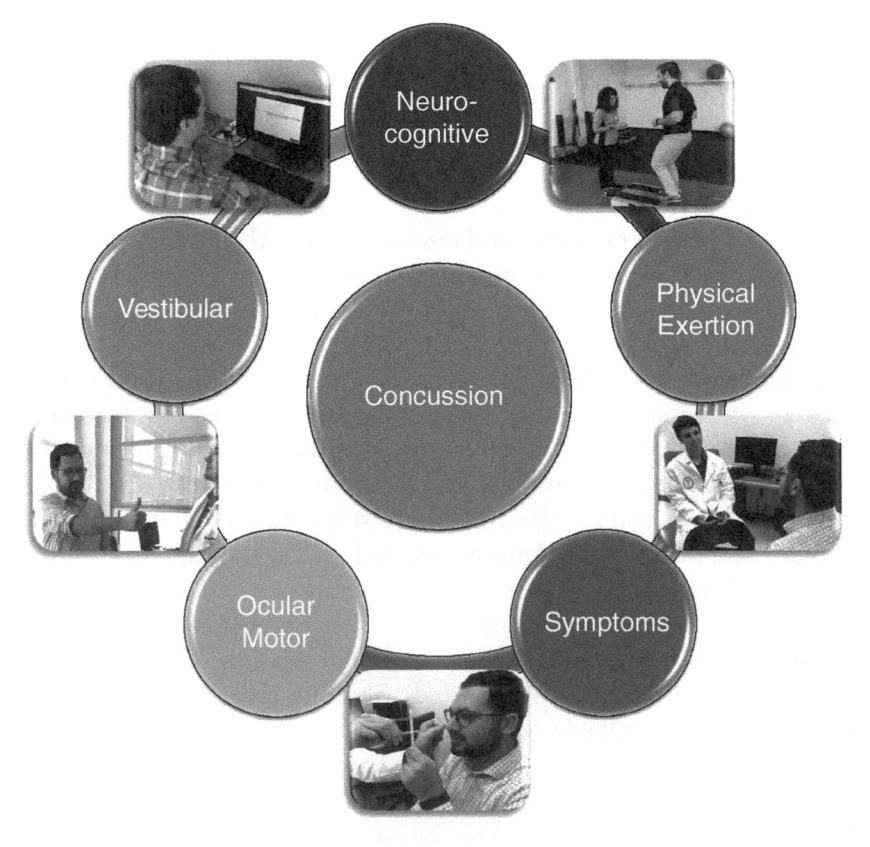

Figure 4.1. Assessment domains for concussion.

As the supporting evidence builds, emerging assessments including blood biomarkers, neuroimaging, and brief screening tools should be incorporated into existing approaches to assess this injury. However, we must avoid assessments that have little empirical evidence behind them. We discuss these emerging assessments later in this chapter. In the sections that follow, we present an approach to conducting a comprehensive clinical assessment for concussion, including acute evaluation at the time of injury, clinical interview, and emerging neuroimaging approaches. The assessments provided herein provide clinicians with the basic tenets of a comprehensive assessment.

ACUTE EVALUATION OF CONCUSSION AT THE TIME OF INJURY

Ideally, concussion assessment begins at the time of injury with an evaluation of the acute presentation of the injury. The information obtained should be communicated to subsequent specialty care and follow-up care providers. Knowledge of the initial concussion characteristics, such as the presence of dizziness (Lau, Kontos, Collins, Mucha, & Lovell, 2011) or post-traumatic amnesia (M. W. Collins et al., 2003), may help predict prognosis and guide initial assessments and subsequent targeted interventions. The acute evaluation may be performed on-field (sport), in theater (military), or on-site (civilian) and conducted by initial care providers such as athletic trainers, corpsmen-level medics, or emergency medical technicians. Emergency and sports medicine physicians may also provide initial evaluation of concussion.

The primary goal of the initial concussion evaluation and care is to assess and triage severe intracranial pathologies as well as cervical spine and other emergent injuries. After ruling out emergent conditions, the initial provider typically conducts a brief concussion assessment. This assessment serves as the foundation for a thorough injury history and provides insight into potential changes in symptoms and impairment since the time of injury. Unfortunately, in many instances, initial care and evaluation of concussion is lacking, and patients seek no initial care and then self-refer to a clinic days or weeks following their injury. In other instances, patients may lack access to appropriate care. In these cases, the patient's self-reported injury history may be the only source of information about the initial characteristics of the concussion.

The initial evaluation of concussion typically consists of (a) injury information; (b) initial signs, symptoms, and severity; (c) orientation to place and time; (d) cognitive function; and (e) balance and motor coordination.

As a result of the potentially adverse outcomes associated with returning to sport and/or military duty following a concussion, it is not surprising that most acute evaluations of concussion emanate from these environments. The Sport Concussion Assessment Tool (SCAT; P. McCrory et al., 2009) is used to assess the five components of an initial evaluation of concussion. (The tool, now in its fourth iteration, is referred to as the SCAT-5 to reflect the number of Concussion in Sport Group meetings in which it was developed and refined; P. McCrory et al., 2017.) The SCAT-5 comprises several different brief assessments, including the Standardized Assessment for Concussion (McCrea et al., 1998), the Balance Error Scoring System (BESS; Guskiewicz, 2001), and the Post-Concussion Symptom Inventory (Gioia, Schneider, Vaughan, & Isquith, 2009), in addition to other neurological and neuromotor assessments of the injury, orientation, and initial signs. The Standardized Assessment for Concussion and its military counterpart, the Military Acute Concussion Evaluation (Defense and Veterans Brain Injury Center, 2012), are commonly used to conduct brief initial cognitive function assessment following concussion. These tools comprise brief tasks of word list and forward and reverse number list (i.e., forwards–backwards digit span) memory that test working and delayed working memories. These tests are useful in detecting cognitive impairment in the initial acute postinjury phase (i.e., within the first few days of the injury; e.g., Barr & McCrea, 2001). The BESS provides a relatively brief (10 minute) clinical assessment of postural stability (Guskiewicz, 2001). For the SCAT-3, a modified version of the BESS was used that included only the three stances performed on the ground, which cut administration time by half. However, the new SCAT-5 has added in the option to complete the entire BESS, which includes three additional stances performed on a compliant foam pad. We discuss the BESS in more detail in the section on balance later in the chapter. The Post-Concussion Symptom Inventory consists of 22 self-reported items and is discussed in the symptom evaluation section later in the chapter.[1]

Although the preceding brief evaluations are important for identifying concussion and documenting initial injury characteristics, they are not without their limitations. In our experience, one of the limitations of these tools, particularly with the Standardized Assessment for Concussion, is a ceiling effect: The test is easy enough that patients can score very high even after sustaining a concussion. In addition, these tests can be found on the Internet, and athletes or military personnel who are motivated to avoid detection often memorize the limited lists of words and numbers on the Standardized Assessment for Concussion and Military Acute Concussion

---

[1]A copy of the SCAT-5 is available at http://bjsm.bmj.com/content/51/11/851. A copy of the child version of the SCAT-5 is available at http://bjsm.bmj.com/content/51/11/862.

Evaluation. Although the BESS detects balance impairment following concussion and may help identify patients with more severe injuries, patients who demonstrate balance impairment typically have multiple impairments and symptoms.

In short, in our experience, the BESS often adds confirmatory data rather than a unique contribution for identifying concussion beyond its acute use on the sideline or at the time of injury. It is easy to administer at the time of injury and can help identify patients in the first couple of days after an injury with vestibulospinal impairment who may benefit from earlier rehabilitation in this area. These tools were also not designed to be used long-term to track recovery beyond the first couple of days following injury (Giza et al., 2013). These acute assessment tools do not assess oculomotor/vision function, vestibular function (beyond balance), and other domains evident at the time of injury. As such, additional acute or time of injury tools that expand these assessment domains are needed.

CLINICAL INTERVIEW: LAYING THE FOUNDATION

The cornerstone of a good clinical evaluation of a patient with concussion is the clinical interview. The purpose of the interview is threefold: (a) establish rapport, trust, and a good therapeutic foundation; (b) uncover detailed injury information; and (c) delve into a patient's personal and familial medical and biopsychosocial history (M. W. Collins, Kontos, Reynolds, Murawski, & Fu, 2014). These three components serve as the foundation for a positive therapeutic relationship and help drive the effectiveness of other assessments.

Therapeutic Relationship

The most critical component to a good clinical interview is developing a strong therapeutic relationship with the patient. The foundational clinical interview skills of building trust, rapport, and empathy are the keys to doing so. However, it is equally important to frame the relationship with the patient in a positive light. Research suggests that contextual framing from health care providers can influence patient outcomes (Mondaini et al., 2007). In fact, our own research suggests that patients who were given specific concussion discharge instructions experienced more symptoms compared with patients who had not received these instructions (Zuckerbraun et al., 2014). Establishing a positive framework reinforced with supportive statements (e.g., "You will recover from this injury," "There are things we can do to get you better") is necessary to promote a positive therapeutic outcome. At the same time, guarantees and timelines for recovery should be avoided, because they can create unrealistic expectations that lead to poor patient outcomes.

Previous patient experiences (especially with previous concussions) should be considered because previous negative outcomes can lead to negative future expectations. It is also important to promote patients' control and active ownership of their recovery to counter potential negative effects from somatic hypervigilance, rumination on symptoms, and withdrawal from normal activities (Heath, 2013).

Concussion has become a bit of a boogeyman—something feared and not well understood. The development of a therapeutic relationship provides opportunity to educate patients about concussion definition, risk factors, concussion types, and treatments. The information in Chapters 1 and 2 can be communicated to the patient during the initial visit to promote better awareness of current injury status and expectations for recovery and treatment. One strategy our clinicians employ is the use of a brain drawing to explain how a concussion occurs, how it affects the brain, and how it leads to symptoms a patient might be experiencing. These pictures of concussion say a thousand words about the injury and help frame a more positive recovery process by eliminating some of the mystery surrounding concussion.

Injury History and Current Injury Information

Injury history can be obtained using a combination of standard intake forms, such as the Ohio State University traumatic brain injury (TBI) history form (Corrigan & Bogner, 2007) and interview questions. It is important to ascertain not only the numbers of previous concussions but also the signs, symptoms, impairment, and dates of each injury. Of particular importance are multiple concussions that occurred over a short period of time; they may represent a single injury that was mismanaged or worsened through multiple impacts. With regard to the current injury, the location and mechanism of injury are critical to understanding the injury and the patient's ability to recall the injury and its effects. Additional relevant information includes initial signs, symptoms, and impairment and any changes in personality, behavior, or mood following the injury. This information should be obtained from the patient, as well as primary caregivers (if the patient is a child) and the initial care provider.

Medical and Biopsychosocial History

Several of the key predictors of poor outcome following concussion are medical history-related factors. For example, personal history and family history of migraine and motion sickness and other vestibular issues are both associated with poor outcomes (Womble et al., 2017). Therefore, obtaining a detailed medical and biopsychosocial history is key to understanding a patient's trajectory following concussion, including likely clinical profiles, severity of symptoms and impairment, and recovery time. In addition, a thorough medical and biopsychosocial history may allow for more targeted and earlier interventions to minimize the effects of the risk factor.

A comprehensive medical and biopsychosocial history includes a variety of components such as personal and family physical (e.g., blood pressure, orthopedic injuries), mental (e.g., depression, anxiety), personal and social (e.g., family, work, school), and substance use (e.g., alcohol, drugs) histories, as well as information about current and previous prescription and over-the-counter medications and supplements. Information about academic (e.g., learning disability, grades) and sport (e.g., type, position, experience) history is also included in a comprehensive medical history, especially for high school- and college-aged and sport populations. Both personal and family histories may provide important information that can influence concussion-related outcomes. Note that a history of diagnosed medical conditions may not be available for younger patients because they may not have been diagnosed. Therefore, if a history of a relevant medical condition, such as migraine, is suspected, the clinician should ask specific questions to determine whether that condition may exist and warrants additional follow-up with an appropriate referral.

SYMPTOM ASSESSMENTS

Symptom assessments are among the most commonly used assessments following a concussion and are recommended by all of the consensus statements and guidelines for assessing concussion (e.g., Giza et al., 2013; P. McCrory et al., 2013). The most common symptom assessment type involves patient self-reported symptoms using a checklist or inventory. Typically, these checklists or inventories assess the number and severity of each symptom, usually on a Likert-type scale of 0 (*none*) to 6 (*severe*) or 0 to 10. There are numerous symptom inventories, including the Graded Symptoms Checklist (Guskiewicz et al., 2004) and Rivermead Post-Concussion Symptom Scale Questionnaire (King, Crawford, Wenden, Moss, & Wade, 1995). One of the most commonly used symptom reports is the Post-Concussion Symptom Scale (Lovell & Collins, 1998). Many of these symptom reports can be found in computerized neurocognitive test batteries (e.g., Post-Concussion Symptom Scale in the Immediate Post-Concussion Assessment and Cognitive Testing [ImPACT]). These embedded symptom reports typically precede the neurocognitive components. However, the timing of these assessments may influence reported symptoms, and so it is advisable to assess symptoms after these tests are administered.

The way in which symptoms are assessed can also affect their reported number and severity (Elbin, Knox, et al., 2016). Symptoms can be assessed through open- or closed-ended interview questions. In addition, symptoms may be reported by other individuals, such as parents, especially for pediatric patients who may lack accuracy or insight into their symptoms following a concussion. Open-ended approaches (e.g., "What symptoms are you currently experiencing") elicit lower total symptom severity scores than closed-ended items. Although parents and children report similar total symptom severity scores using closed-ended items (Elbin, Knox, et al., 2016), parents tend to report more observable symptoms, such as changes in mood, sleep, and behavior. In contrast, parents may be less aware of somatic symptoms because they are less observable. Research suggests that symptom reporting may be influenced by the way in which symptom items are presented. For example, if symptom items are presented with the most common symptoms clustered together, overall symptoms—both number endorsed and total symptom severity scores—tended to be higher (Kwan, Wojcik, Miron-Shatz, Votruba, & Olivola, 2012). Similarly, presenting symptom items using a negative preface such as, "Check all of the items you are not currently experiencing," may result in lower symptom scores (C. Olivola, personal communication, March 1, 2016). Therefore, consistent timing and approach in assessing symptoms is important to ensure that changes in symptoms are accurately reflected.

Patients often report headache or dizziness as a symptom. Both have numerous subtypes and involve various etiologies. Headaches may be pressure, cluster, migraine, ocular-migraine, or medication-rebound in origin. Dizziness may be vestibular, cervicogenic, migraine-related, or from some other cause. Consequently, additional assessments of symptom subtypes provide a better understanding of the etiology and specific characteristics of certain symptoms. We recently developed a visual analog scale, the Headache Electronic Diary for Children With Concussion, to assess headache pain following a concussion in children that can be used in children as young as 5 years old (Pasek et al., 2015). This and similar measures allow more in-depth monitoring and investigation of the nature of specific headache and related symptoms.

Assessing symptoms in the pediatric age group is challenging because children generally lack insight into concussion symptoms and understanding of terminology used to describe symptoms. Researchers have suggested that children are better at reporting internalized (somatic) symptoms but worse at reporting externalized (cognitive) symptoms than adults (Hodges, Gordon, & Lennon, 1990; Rey, Schrader, & Morris-Yates, 1992). Therefore, specific age-appropriate symptom inventories are used with younger patients; usually this means "ask their parents/guardians." The SCAT-5 Child is an example of a pediatric-specific symptom report that relies on parent/guardian reporting of symptoms (P. McCrory et al., 2017). Instead of using specific symptom reports, some clinicians may want to use a perceived pain (i.e., Borg) or similar semantic-based scale. These scales may be more useful in determining the overall severity of symptoms following a concussion than determining which specific symptoms a young patient is experiencing.

Although some patients may underreport symptoms because they lack insight into or understanding about concussion symptoms, others may purposefully minimize their symptoms to return to sport, military service, or other activities. In our experience, both elite athletes and Special Operations Forces personnel with concussion may underreport symptoms to expedite return to sport or duty, respectively. In contrast, some patients overreport symptoms. Overreporting may result from somaticizing or reporting high levels of vague symptoms regardless of injury or illness (Root et al., 2016). Other patients may exaggerate or conflate their symptoms because they are malingering. Patients who are in litigation, who claim worker's compensation, and who may have other tangible gains from their concussion may also malinger (see Chapter 3). As such, symptom reports must be taken with a grain of salt and should be corroborated with additional information based on observation, patient behavior, others' reports and observations, and other assessments including computerized neurocognitive and vestibular/ oculomotor testing.

Excessive monitoring and reporting of symptoms following concussion may lead to patients dwelling on or overanalyzing their symptoms such that they report more symptoms. In our experience, patients who somaticize are more likely to fixate on their symptoms. Therefore, we recommend symptom evaluation or reporting no more than once or twice a week following concussion and after the initial interview.

NEUROCOGNITIVE ASSESSMENTS

Neurocognitive assessments are commonly used to assess concussion, particularly sport- and recreation-related concussion (Kontos, Sufrinko, Womble, & Kegel, 2016). Nearly 70% of sports medicine staff reportedly use these assessments (R. M. Williams, Welch, Weber, Parsons, & Valovich McLeod, 2014). Unfortunately, these tests are often erroneously believed to represent quintessential "concussion tests," and if patients pass them, then they are no longer concussed. In reality, these assessments represent a key tool in a comprehensive approach to assessing concussion that also includes symptoms, balance, and vestibular and oculomotor assessments. Neurocognitive assessments may be conducted using paper-and-pencil or computerized versions. Although computerized versions of these tests are more frequently used for concussion, we first discuss the paper-and-pencil assessments from which the computerized versions were developed.

Paper-and-Pencil Assessments

Paper-and-pencil tests cover cognitive domains of intelligence, learning, attention, and processing speed. These tests can be broad and include subtest batteries (e.g., Repeatable Battery for the Assessment of Neuropsychological Status; Randolph, 1998), or they can have specific and narrow focus on a single cognitive domain (e.g., language in the Boston Naming Test; Goodglass, Kaplan, & Weintraub, 2001). Summaries of commonly used paper-and-pencil tests and their concomitant domains are available in our article focusing on neuropsychological assessment in concussion (see Kontos, Sufrinko, Womble, & Kegel, 2016). In addition to cognitive domains, effort-based tests determine whether patients commit full effort during testing and detect malingering.

Paper-and-pencil tests are lengthy, require a licensed psychology professional for interpretation, and suffer from a lack of availability of preinjury performance (Iverson & Schatz, 2015). Nonetheless, such tests help clinicians probe deeply into a specific cognitive domain to augment computerized neurocognitive test results. However, these tests do not fit into the briefer models of patient care that predominate health care.

Computerized Assessments

Computerized neurocognitive tests (CNTs) are among the most commonly used subacute assessment following concussion. These tests typically measure performance on attention, memory, reaction time, and processing speed tasks. These tests were developed in the late 1990s when personal computers became more powerful and accessible. CNTs offer several advantages over paper-and-pencil tests: (a) speed of completion (20–30 minutes completion time); (b) ability to administer the tests to multiple individuals at one time; (c) random, multiple forms limit practice effects and allow for serial testing; and (d) accurate measurement of reaction time. As a result of these advantages, CNTs are widely used to assess concussion, particularly sport- and recreation-related concussions (Kontos, Sufrinko, Womble, & Kegel, 2016).

Baseline Testing

Ideally, a preinjury (baseline) level of cognitive performance is obtained through baseline testing. This approach has been used since CNTs first started being used in the 1990s (Wojtys et al., 1999). Postinjury performance is compared with baseline performance to determine the extent of cognitive domain impairment following a concussion. Baseline testing may be available through concussion outreach efforts, such as the Heads Up Pittsburgh outreach initiative in Pittsburgh, Pennsylvania, which is funded in part by the Pittsburgh Penguins Foundation affiliated with the Pittsburgh Penguins from the National Hockey League (see Chapter 5). This program provides reduced cost or free baseline neurocognitive testing to patients in addition to awareness and education to patients and their families. These tests typically cost $15 to $25 each and often provide concussion education and awareness programming. Baseline testing may also be completed as part of mandated state- or school board-legislated concussion protocols.

Group administration of computerized neurocognitive baseline tests has been criticized by some as an invalid approach that leads to inaccurate baseline scores (Moser, Schatz, Neidzwski, & Ott, 2011). However, more recent evidence suggests no differences between individual and group administrations of adolescents and children (Vaughan, Gerst, Sady, Newman, & Gioia, 2014). Kuhn and Solomon (2014) reported that unsupervised student-athletes performed worse on baseline tests than a supervised cohort. Other researchers have intimated concerns of purposely scoring low on baseline neurocognitive testing, particularly in sport settings (Erdal, 2012). However, data indicate that purposely scoring low (sandbagging) on a baseline is quite difficult. In fact, 100% of test takers instructed to purposefully sandbag baseline tests were identified using validity markers (Schatz & Glatts, 2013). In lieu of baseline testing, clinicians can use published normative values for age and gender groups to assess postconcussion impairment. However, use of normative values for CNTs should take into consideration the role of factors that influence test performance.

Postconcussion Testing

To assess cognitive function following a concussion, CNTs offer several advantages over paper-and-pencil approaches, including faster administration, decreased scoring and interpretation time, lower cost, and more accurate reaction time measures (Kontos, Sufrinko, Womble, & Kegel, 2016). Several CNTs are commonly used to assess concussion, including Automated Neurocognitive Assessment Metric (Levinson & Reeves, 1997), Axon Sports Computerized Cognitive Assessment Tool (Collie, Maruff, Darby, & McStephen, 2003; Falleti, Maruff, Collie, & Darby, 2006), Concussion Vital Signs (n.d.), Head Minder CRI (Erlanger, Feldman, et al., 2003), and the Immediate Post-Concussion Assessment and Cognitive Testing (ImPACT; ImPACT Applications, Inc., Pittsburgh, Pennsylvania). These tests typically include components that focus on memory, attention, processing speed, and reaction time. However, some of the tests may be weighted more heavily on one component or another. For example, CogSport includes predominantly reaction time tasks. As a result of this weighting, clinicians should be cognizant of the individual tasks that compose a CNT and augment as needed with additional testing to represent a breadth of cognitive domains. Again, published normative values for CNTs can be used when available to allow for postinjury interpretation in the absence of a premorbid baseline. Normative values are limited by age (11–50-year-olds).

Not all CNTs are equally effective in assessing cognitive deficits following concussion. In fact, in a meta-analysis, we found that memory detected impairment following concussion better than reaction time (Kontos, Braithwaite, Dakan, & Elbin, 2014).

Factors That Influence Performance on Computerized Neurocognitive Tests

Several factors may influence performance on CNTs. Most important, clinicians should ensure that a patient's performance on a CNT is valid (Schatz, Moser, Solomon, Ott, & Karpf, 2012). A combination of procedural error (e.g., allowing parents to assist children with the test), environmental factors (e.g., noise, distractions), and varying levels of effort may influence performance on the tests. Consequently, it is important to follow carefully test manufacturers' directions for administering these tests and gauge effort using one or more tests of effort such as the Medical Symptom Validity Test developed by neuropsychologist Paul Green (2004).

Researchers have reported that sleep can affect both baseline (Sufrinko, Johnson, & Henry, 2016) and postinjury (Sufrinko, Pearce, et al., 2015) performance on CNTs. Some researchers have argued that both the amount and quality of sleep on the night preceding the administration of a test (McClure, Zuckerman, Kutscher, Gregory, & Solomon, 2014) and an individual's general sleep hygiene (Mihalik et al., 2013) may adversely affect neurocognitive performance. Some individual test components, such as the motor processing speed test on ImPACT, may have more pronounced learning or test effects, such that improvements in performance might obscure clinically relevant findings.

Criticisms of Computerized Neurocognitive Tests

During the past decade, several groups of researchers (e.g., Alsalaheen, Stockdale, Pechumer, & Broglio, 2016; Broglio, Macciocchi, & Ferrara, 2007; Mayers & Redick, 2012; Randolph, 2011) have criticized CNTs as being unreliable and of limited value in assessing and managing concussion. However, these criticisms have applied different standards to CNTs than have other assessments (Schatz et al., 2012). Moreover, these studies were characterized by one or more of the following: (a) unsupported generalizations, (b) selective reporting/inclusion of data or studies, (c) misapplication of statistical approaches to reliability (particularly test–retest reliability), and (d) a limited perspective of validity (Schatz et al., 2012).

In fact, test–retest reliability for other commonly used tools to assess concussion shows that the reliability of CNTs is often higher than those reported for other measures. Specifically, test–retest reliability of these tests was higher, ranging from 0.46 to 0.76, whereas the test–retest reliability of clinical balance (i.e., BESS) was between 0.57 and 0.60 and brief cognitive tools (i.e., Standardized Assessment for Concussion) was 0.46. For comparison, research involving physiological measures such as ambulatory blood pressure reports test–retest reliability of $r = 0.84–0.88$ for systolic blood pressure and $r = 0.83–0.86$ diastolic blood pressure (Cornish, Blanchard, & Jaccard, 1995). Recently, we reexamined the reliability of one CNT, ImPACT, and reported that test–retest is dependent not only on the statistics used but also on the timing between assessments and other factors such as age and gender (Womble, Reynolds, Schatz, Shah, & Kontos, 2016). Therefore, clinicians must scrutinize published reviews and empirical papers to make sure they are comparable and provide complete data. (For a thorough review of the evidence behind CNTs, see Kontos, Sufrinko, Womble, & Kegel, 2016.)

NEUROMOTOR ASSESSMENTS

Following a concussion, patients may experience a number of neuromotor deficits such as balance or walking difficulty, trouble integrating sensory information, and dizziness and vertigo symptoms (Kontos & Ortega, 2011). Researchers and clinicians have developed a variety of measures, predominately focused on balance, to assess neuromotor effects following concussion. However, balance measures only assess postural stability in static or dynamic conditions. Therefore, other measures, such as gait and vestibular and oculomotor assessments, are warranted. Moreover, these additional assessments help to inform clinical profiles and referrals for subsequent targeted therapeutic interventions. Finally, the return to activity, play, or duty approach advocated in this book and in consensus statements necessitates a comprehensive screening of neuromotor deficits and symptoms (M. W. Collins, Kontos, et al., 2014; P. McCrory et al., 2013). A comprehensive screening should include assessments of balance, gait, and vestibular/oculomotor domains.

Balance

Two primary measures are used to assess balance following concussion: clinical balance assessments and force plate–based assessments. The former are easy to implement and require little equipment but rely on subjective test administrator interpretation or scoring of performance errors with limited reliability. The latter require expensive equipment and considerable time and space to administer, but provide a highly valid and reliable assessment of postural control or balance.

Clinical Balance Assessments

The most commonly used clinical balance measure is the BESS (Guskiewicz, 2001), which involves a series of three stances (double leg, single leg, tandem) performed for 20 seconds with eyes closed and arms placed on the hips on solid ground and on a foam balance pad. A modified version is now available and reduces administration time while maintaining similar validity to the full version (Hunt, Ferrara, Bornstein, & Baumgartner, 2009). The modified version involves three stances without the pad. In both versions, a trained observer scores errors and evaluates performance. The BESS is based on the Romberg test (Rogers, 1980; Roy & Irvin, 1983), which represents a more simplified (i.e., one stance) clinical balance screening test.

The BESS is effective at measuring balance deficits during the first few days postinjury (Giza et al., 2013). The utility of the BESS and similar measures declines 3 days after the injury (McCrea et al., 2003). In response to this criticism, some researchers have applied concurrent videogame and accelerometer-based assessments to the BESS to provide more objectivity to the evaluation (e.g., N. Murray, Salvatore, Powell, & Reed-Jones, 2014). There also are concerns about practice effects associated with repeated BESS administrations (Valovich, Perrin, & Gansneder, 2003). Additional research on these measures is needed before they can be used clinically to evaluate balance following a concussion. Although the BESS is useful in assessing balance impairment in the acute and early subacute postinjury phase, it cannot identify the source of the abhorrent signal that results in impaired balance. Given that balance impairment could stem from disruptions to both afferent (sensory) and efferent (motor) neuronal pathways, additional balance tests that can make this determination should be applied when assessing concussion.

Force Plate–Based Balance Assessments

The other approach to measuring balance following concussion is the force plate–based assessment. This approach involves using a portable or in-ground force plate to measure sway in anterior–posterior and medial–lateral directions, as well as center of pressure and center of mass during the performance of balance. The most commonly used force plate measure is the Sensory Organization Test (NeuroCom, Inc., Clackamas, Oregon). Like the BESS, the Sensory Organization Test involves a series of six conditions lasting 20 seconds. However, unlike the BESS, the Sensory Organization Test conditions involve both eyes opened and closed conditions and a combination of tilted platform and tilted visual field conditions. These tests allow the test administrator to determine whether imbalance is due to disruption of somatosensory or visual/vestibular function. Similarly, the Clinical Test of Sensory Integration and Balance (Ingersoll & Armstrong, 1992; Shumway-Cook & Horak, 1986) measures center of mass and center of pressure, which are more sensitive to perturbation in balance but require sophisticated equipment, including motion capture cameras and force plates that are not widely available.

Other Balance Assessments

Recently, several more accessible assessments of balance have appeared in the marketplace and in research papers. Many of these approaches take advantage of native accelerometer-based technology available in most smartphones. These accelerometers are the same ones that allow us to play driving and other movement-based videogames on our phones. One example of these other balance assessments is the Sway Balance (see http://swaymedical.com) program, an online application using accelerometer technology to measure anterior–posterior and medial–lateral sway while subjects hold a tablet or smartphone. These new tools are inexpensive and accessible, but they lack empirical evidence at this time.

Gait

In contrast to balance assessments, gait assessments are used less frequently to assess concussion. However, assessing gait may play an important role in concussion assessment, particularly for patients with vestibular and oculomotor clinical profiles. Additionally, the evidence for decreases in gait performance following concussion is growing (Fino, Nussbaum, & Brolinson, 2016; Oldham, Munkasy, Evans, Wikstrom, & Buckley, 2016). Two primary clinical assessments of gait are used following concussion: the Functional Gait Assessment (FGA: Wrisley, Marchetti, Kuharsky, & Whitney, 2004) and its predecessor, the Dynamic Gait Index (DGI: Shumway-Cook & Woollacott, 1995). These two assessments are similar and comprise a series of walking movements during the performance of head turns. The 10-item FGA assesses the subject's ability to walk with head turns, changes of speed, and around obstacles. Similar to the FGA, the eight-item DGI measures gait during the performance of dynamic movements including stepping around obstacles, changing gait speeds, and with head movements. The DGI is similar to the FGA but has several distinct movements. Higher scores on both tests indicate normal gait. In our clinical experience, most patients who have had a concussion perform at or near the maximum score on these assessments. However, patients with vestibular and oculomotor clinical profiles tend to perform poorly or provoke symptoms during these assessments. As such, gait assessments can play a role in a comprehensive concussion assessment.

More advanced assessments of gait, including those using high-speed motion capture cameras and biomechanical light markers, are employed in the research laboratory setting. However, these types of assessments require specialized, expensive equipment and do not currently provide clinically useful outcomes. Moreover, they require larger spaces to measure gait.

Vestibular and Oculomotor Assessments

Recent findings highlight the importance of assessing vestibular and oculomotor domains following concussion (Mucha et al., 2014; Sussman, Ho, Pendharkar, & Ghajar, 2016). We developed a systematic brief screening tool for this purpose. In short, we wanted a tool to screen patients who might need additional, in-depth testing and referral for targeted vestibular and/or oculomotor treatments. The culmination of over a decade of clinical insight working with patients with concussion, together with expert input from vestibular and physical therapy experts, led to the development of what was initially referred to as the Vestibular Screening Form. For 5 years, this form was tested on patients, expanded to include oculomotor components, honed to be more parsimonious, and renamed the Vestibular/Ocular Motor Screening (VOMS; Mucha et al., 2014).

The VOMS can be implemented as one component of a comprehensive assessment of concussion to measure vestibular and oculomotor symptoms and impairment. The tool is a short (5–7 minute) clinical screening assessment that can help identify patients with vestibular and oculomotor impairment and symptoms who may need subsequent testing and referral for targeted treatment and rehabilitation. The only equipment the test requires is a visual fixation stick and a Gulick anthropometric tape measure. The VOMS consists of five test domains: (a) smooth pursuits, (b) horizontal and vertical saccades, (c) Near Point of Convergence (NPC; a measure of the proximity of a fixation target to the nose while maintaining fusion, i.e., prior to the image doubling), (d) horizontal and vertical vestibulo-ocular reflex (VOR), and (e) visual motion sensitivity (see Figure 4.2).

The VOMS begins with an assessment of headache, fogginess, dizziness, and nausea symptoms prior to the administration of the test. Each symptom is rated on a scale of 0 (*none*) to 10 (*very high*). Approximately 10 seconds after the visual motion sensitivity and VOR components of the VOMS and immediately following all other components, patients report on symptoms again to determine whether any component provoked symptoms. In addition, the VOMS includes three measurements of NPC distance in centimeters that

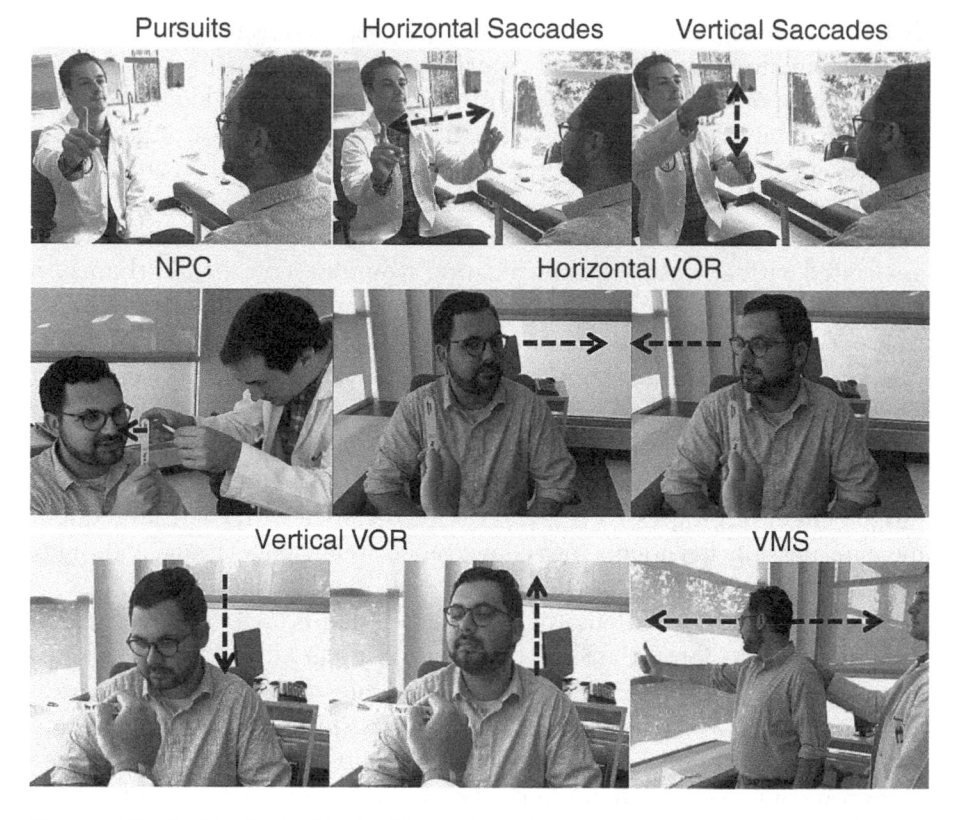

Figure 4.2. The Vestibular/Ocular Motor Screening tool includes assessments of (a) smooth pursuits, (b) horizontal and vertical saccades, (c) near point convergence, (d) horizontal and vertical vestibulo-ocular reflex, and (e) visual motion sensitivity.

are averaged across the three trials. The NPC distance is measured from the distance at which the fixation stick splits into two images as reported by the patient to the tip of the nose.

Preliminary evidence for the VOMS indicates that the tool is both internally consistent and useful in identifying concussed from matched healthy controls (Mucha et al., 2014). We also found two clinical cutoff levels for the VOMS: a symptom score of greater than or equal to 2 on any single VOMS item, and average near point convergence (NPC) distance of greater than or equal to 5 centimeters. Using these clinical cutoff levels, we increased our ability to distinguish concussed from matched healthy controls compared with chance alone by 38% (NPC distance = 5+ centimeters) and 50% (single VOMS item symptom score = 2+). Our research also suggests that very few healthy, uninjured individuals report any symptoms at either baseline or following each of the VOMS components (Mucha et al.,

2014). However, certain modifying risk factors, such as female sex, a history of migraine headaches, and especially motion sickness, may influence performance on the VOMS among otherwise healthy individuals (Kontos, Sufrinko, Elbin, Puskar, & Collins, 2016). As such, clinicians should account for these factors when interpreting baseline VOMS symptoms scores.

In a current study that is under review, we have found that sex, on-field dizziness, and subacute posttraumatic migraine and fogginess are all associated with at least one clinical cutoff symptom score greater than 2 on the VOMS (Womble et al., 2017). Findings from our recent study indicate that patients with NPC distance of greater than or equal to 5 centimeters (i.e., convergence insufficiency) scored worse on verbal memory, visual motor speed, and reaction time (Pearce, Sufrinko, et al., 2015). These patients also reported more concussion symptoms than did patients with normal NPC distance less than 5 centimeters. We also reported tentative support for a fatigue effect of progressively greater NPC distance with each subsequent measure, but only in patients with convergence insufficiency (Pearce, Sufrinko, et al., 2015).

Another test of oculomotor performance that is used to assess patients following concussion is the King-Devick (Galetta et al., 2011) test, a timed test of saccadic eye movements that was originally designed for use to assess attention deficit and related disorders. The King-Devick test comprises four cards, including one practice card and three test cards. The cards include eight rows of five single-digit numbers each. Patients read the lines from left to right as quickly and accurately as possible. Completion time and errors are recorded and then compared with a patient's baseline performance (Galetta et al., 2011) or normative data (Rizzo et al., 2016) if a baseline is unavailable. Initial evidence suggests the King-Devick is useful in measuring impairment in saccadic eye movement following concussion (Seidman et al., 2015). However, performance on the King-Devick may be influenced by practice effects, resulting in potential false negatives (King, Hume, Gissane, & Clark, 2015).

Recent research has questioned the use of the King-Devick test to detect concussion in the emergency department setting (Silverberg, Luoto, Öhman, & Iverson, 2014). Although the test may provide a useful assessment of saccadic eye movements, it does not assess other components of oculomotor function and does not include vestibular components. The King-Devick test also does not assess symptom provocation following performance of the test. As such, it may provide an objective assessment of timed saccadic eye movements, but it does not assess other areas of oculomotor and vestibular impairment or symptoms. The King-Devick may be best used in conjunction with the VOMS and other tests to screen for vestibular and oculomotor impairment and symptoms following concussion.

PSYCHOLOGICAL ASSESSMENTS

Psychological issues often become apparent following concussion (Kontos, Deitrick, & Reynolds, 2016). Consequently, the use of brief psychological assessments to screen patients following concussion may help identify patients experiencing mood, anxiety, stress, and other emotional issues. However, brief psychological screening tools are not commonly used as part of a standard assessment approach with patients who sustain concussion. Also, in-depth psychological evaluation and referrals may be warranted depending on the results of initial screening. As for patients with a suspected psychological disorder, assessment begins with a thorough psychological history and mental status exam and interview. Such an approach should include an in-depth history of personal and family psychological and related issues. In addition, evaluations of sleep, behavior change, mood, medication, family, substance use, and suicide ideation are indicated following concussion. Injury-specific information about the patient's concussion including pain, headache, dizziness/vertigo, and the effect of the injury on occupational/academic and social functioning should also be evaluated.

Other commonly used assessment approaches may involve self-report inventories consisting of both psychological and neuropsychological test batteries. As a starting point, clinicians should employ brief screening tools such as the Patient Health Questionnaire–9 (Kroenke, Spitzer, & Williams, 2001), which measures depression or general anxiety. Additional screening tools, such as the Alcohol Use Disorder Identification Test (Babor, de la Fuente, Saunders, & Grant, 1992), may be warranted for patients with potential substance use issues following concussion. In support of this screening, limited research has suggested a link between concussion and substance abuse; additional empirical studies are needed to better understand this link (Finkbeiner, Max, Longman, & Debert, 2016). If any of the screening tools or the clinical interview identifies potential psychological issues, then more in-depth assessment and documentation involving inventories and potential referrals are warranted. Among the more commonly used inventories are the Brief Symptom Inventory (Derogatis, 1993), which assesses a variety of mood-related symptoms, and the Profile of Mood States (McNair, Lorr, & Droppleman, 1981), which measures a variety of affective areas, including anger, anxiety, confusion, depression, fatigue, and vigor. More specific measures such as the Beck Depression Inventory (second edition; Beck, Steer, & Brown, 1996) and the Beck Anxiety Inventory (Beck, Epstein, Brown, & Steer, 1988) may also be used for in-depth assessment of specific psychological issues.

Additional measures such as somatization scales like the Children Somatization Inventory (Walker, Beck, Garber, & Lambert, 2009) may also be useful, especially with pediatric populations (Root et al., 2016). It is important to note that age and developmental-specific measures should be employed whenever available to ensure valid assessments. Some researchers have advocated for psychophysiological assessments such as electromyography, electroencephalogram, and heart rate and blood pressure measures (Conder & Conder, 2015). With the increased availability of fitness tracker devices, some clinicians have begun using these assessments to track everything from physical activity to sleep and nutrition. However, at the current time, there is little evidence to support the use of these approaches to assess psychological issues following concussion; these measures should be used in combination with more established approaches.

A final note regarding assessment: When assessing concussion in sport and military populations, baseline psychological evaluations can go a long way toward helping clinicians determine preinjury levels of psychological health. As such, we recommend baseline psychological assessments for athletes and military personnel whenever practical (Covassin, Elbin, Larson, & Kontos, 2012).

EXERTION-BASED ASSESSMENTS

Exertion-based assessments for concussion have been used over the past decade to determine safe return to play and active duty in sport and military populations (P. McCrory et al., 2005). However, it was not until recently that exertion-based assessments began to be used by clinicians to assist in the initial evaluation of patients with concussion (Leddy, Baker, Kozlowski, Bisson, & Willer, 2011). Most of the research on exertion-based assessments has focused on adults (Leddy et al., 2011), and these types of assessments are typically employed several weeks after an injury (Dematteo et al., 2015; Kozlowski, Graham, Leddy, Devinney-Boymel, & Willer, 2013). In our clinical experience, low to moderate intensity exertion-based assessments can be safely used earlier (1–2 weeks postinjury) in the recovery process. Higher intensity exertion should not be used, and clinicians should pay close attention to symptom provocation during any exertion-based assessment. In addition, exertion testing can be conducted with minimal equipment and space, although trained physical therapists should always supervise any exertion-based assessments. For example, simple step tests for aerobic exertion can be conducted in a small clinic office with minimal equipment, and dynamic exertion testing can be conducted in a relatively small hallway or open area or even outside given the right weather and environment.

Aerobic Exertion

Recent evidence suggests that aerobic exertion may be a useful tool to not only assess recovery following concussion (Kozlowski et al., 2013) but also improve symptoms (Dematteo et al., 2015). Silverberg and colleagues (2016) demonstrated that physical activity in the first 10 days following a concussion does not provoke symptom increases in pediatric patients, which suggests that exertion is safe at this time. In a small study of 54 youth with postconcussion syndrome several months after a concussion, researchers found that 63% of patients reported symptoms during exertion (Dematteo et al., 2015). Symptoms, especially cognitive and psychological symptoms, such as feeling nervous, sad, or emotional, generally improved 30 minutes to 24 hours following aerobic exertion; however, some increases in symptoms with exertion were noted. This finding is not surprising given that exercise improves mood (e.g., Carter, Morres, Meade, & Callaghan, 2016) and enhances attention (Vanhelst et al., 2016). Moreover, vestibular-related symptoms increased and did not abate until 24 hours later, suggesting that the aerobic exertion provoked these symptoms more other symptoms. Therefore, clinicians should avoid using exertion protocols with every patient as a routine practice; instead, they should focus on matching appropriate exertion protocols to concussion clinical profiles.

Although aerobic exertion-based assessments are important and may help detect symptoms and deficits that are related to cerebrovascular dysfunction, they need to be complemented with dynamic exertion protocols. With that in mind, a combination of aerobic and dynamic exertion protocols is needed to assess patients following concussion.

Dynamic Exertion

With regard to concussion, exertion typically has been conceptualized as aerobic in nature, focusing on static, heart rate-based exertion, such as stationary cycling and treadmill running. However, sports, military, and many daily activities require body movements where the head and body must move dynamically in concert. These dynamic movements may include lateral movements, movements that involve coordinating head and body movements, integration of visual input, and proprioceptive awareness and navigation. In short, dynamic movements are requisites, and the use of dynamic exertion helps in concussion assessment. For example, after a concussion a hockey player may have no symptoms while running on a treadmill but experience significant symptoms during lateral movements that closely mimic hockey play. Any dynamic exertion assessment following concussion should focus on symptom provocation following each activity, similar to the approach with aerobic exertion.

Unfortunately, no studies have examined the role of dynamic exertion in assessing concussion. One reason for this lack of research is that dynamic exertion is typically tailored to reflect the environment to which each patient will return following concussion. For example, returning to physical education classes requires different dynamic movements than does returning to long-distance truck driving or playing point in basketball. As such, there is no single, comprehensive protocol for dynamic exertion that can be used with all patients. Instead, exertion activities are individualized. We believe that a combination of lateral whole-body and head movements is required to mimic real-life (e.g., driving, playing sport, military performance) movements that may provoke symptoms. Without such assessments, clinicians may miss provocation-based symptoms and impairments that patients may experience later and erroneously attribute to causes other than their concussion, resulting in prolonged recovery from concussion.

EMERGING ASSESSMENTS

There is no shortage of "concussion tests" available. In fact, a summer 2017 Google search of "concussion test" returned more than 3,490,000 results! The current state of the marketplace for products to diagnose concussion has been likened to the snake oil salesmen of the 1800s, complete with grandiose promises and limited or no evidence supporting claims. Despite claims to the contrary, no current U.S. Food and Drug Administration (FDA)–approved single, diagnostic test for concussion is available. However, in summer 2016, ImPACT Applications, Inc., received "de novo" FDA approval for the ImPACT test as a concussion-specific assessment. This is the first company and test to receive this designation, and it may have opened the door for other companies seeking this product designation. Another company, Anthro Tronix, Inc., successfully obtained FDA approval for its product, Defense Automated Neurobehavioral Assessment, for use as a TBI (not concussion specific) diagnosis tool.

In the meantime, gaps in the current assessments used for concussion have resulted in a variety of emerging approaches. Among the more promising of these assessments for concussion are neuroimaging and blood biomarker approaches. While blood biomarkers for concussion represent a fairly recent (i.e., the past decade) development in the field, neuroimaging approaches have been used with varying degrees of success for several decades. Similarly, dual task paradigms, which involve using two or more competing tests (e.g., balance and cognitive) have seen a growth in research and clinical application over the past decade. These approaches are described in the sections that follow.

Dual Task Assessments

Preliminary evidence indicates that dual task paradigms involving a combined assessment of gait or balance and a cognitive task may be an effective approach to assess concussion and its effects (Register-Mihalik, Littleton, & Guskiewicz, 2013). However, more research is needed before these dual tasks can become part of a standard clinical concussion assessment. These paradigms are based on the notion that current approaches to assessment after a concussion focus on one task or domain, which can allow for compensatory strategies to be successful; a depleted brain can reorganize to perform a single task.

However, not all dual task paradigms are the same. In fact, dual task combinations that are fairly easy to perform may actually result in increased balance performance in healthy individuals (Broglio, Tomporowski, & Ferrara, 2005). Therefore, more complex cognitive tasks have been advanced (Howell, Osternig, Koester, & Chou, 2014). This paradoxical finding may result from shifting attention away from an automatic task (balance), where it may have unintended effects of decreasing performance, toward the cognitive task, thereby allowing for a more automatic performance of balance. The key is to present the brain with a sufficiently challenging dual task paradigm that negates compensatory strategies. To that end, we are currently conducting research to determine the effectiveness of a novel, cognitive-balance dual task to assess vestibular impairment following concussion. Our initial findings suggest that performance of a specific component of a visual reaction time task involving an inhibition of response is particularly problematic among concussed patients compared with healthy controls (Kontos, Woolford, et al., 2016). Although this finding is promising, it and previously reported findings should be expanded before dual task paradigms become a standard component of concussion assessment.

Neuroimaging Approaches

Concussions are often referred to as functional injuries that are seemingly "invisible" (Bloom, Horton, McCrory, & Johnston, 2004; Kontos, Collins, & Russo, 2004). However, it is more likely that available neuroimaging approaches are not sensitive enough to detect the subtle changes in the brain associated with concussion. Moreover, concussion stems from underlying structural changes involving diffused axonal injury and contusion, but it also involves functional and neurometabolic changes (Giza & Hovda, 2001; P. McCrory et al., 2013) that may not be evident in standard structural neuroimaging such as computerized tomography (CT) and magnetic resonance imaging (MRI). Therefore, it is likely that a combined structural, functional, and metabolic suite of neuroimaging will yield the best approach to "seeing" concussion and help corroborate clinical assessments of the various clinical profiles of concussion. Current approaches to neuroimaging following concussion focus on identifying global findings across all patients, despite clinical evidence that suggests we should look for specific evidence to support each clinical profile. After all, if two patients have different clinical presentations, wouldn't we expect that the underlying changes in the brain might differ as well?

Standard Structural Neuroimaging With CT and MRI

Currently, no accepted clinical neuroimaging protocol for concussion is available. Researchers use CT and MRI to identify damage in the brain following concussion, with limited results (Bazarian, Blyth, & Cimpello, 2006). CT scanning involves a combination of multiple X-ray images and computerized mapping of the brain to examine structural damage, including skull fractures and bleeding. Because a CT scan uses multiple X-rays to construct the images of the brain, the exposure to radiation is higher than with standard X-rays, and its use should be limited with children (Brenner & Hall, 2007). In addition, CT scans may involve an injected dye contrast to allow for better imaging of the brain resulting in an invasive procedure compared with other imaging approaches. In contrast, MRI is noninvasive and uses powerful magnets together with radio waves to image damage to soft tissue structures of the brain, including changes in volume and lesions.

These techniques were designed to assess more severe damage to the brain, including skull fractures and bleeding (e.g., subdural hematoma), as opposed to the subtle effects of concussion and are not clinically indicated for concussion (Davis et al., 2009; Yuh et al., 2014). Standard clinical neuroimaging with CT scanning and MRI is negative (i.e., no abnormal findings) in a majority (90%–95%) of patients with concussion; therefore, they should be avoided as diagnostic tools for concussion (Pulsipher et al., 2011). Any diagnostic yield from conventional CT scanning and MRI for patients with concussion is minimal and not worth the concomitant risks (Morgan et al., 2015).

Functional Magnetic Resonance Imaging

Researchers have used functional magnetic resonance imaging (fMRI) for some time to evaluate functional changes in blood flow using blood oxygen level dependent (BOLD) signal associated with the performance of task paradigms, such as memory tasks. Findings from fMRI research suggest that BOLD signals are reduced in patients after a concussion (e.g., Lovell et al., 2007). Other research has focused on resting state fMRI, which is more practical from a clinical perspective because it does not require as much time and limits some of the imaging noise associated with the performance paradigm-based fMRI tasks (e.g., Czerniak et al., 2015). However, fMRI evaluation requires expensive and sensitive equipment not typically available outside of academic medical and research centers. In summary, fMRI provides a noninvasive assessment of metabolic function and can be used at rest and during performance of certain tasks, but it is expensive, time-consuming, involves lots of loud noises for patients that may exacerbate symptoms, and currently has limited clinical utility.

Diffusion Tensor Imaging

Diffusion tensor imaging (DTI), which assesses white matter tracts and the integrity of fiber structures by measuring the direction and flow of water molecules, may provide a better imaging alternative to conventional MRI. The two primary measures of white matter tract damage or integrity used in DTI are fractional anisotropy (FA), which measures the directional nature of water molecules, and mean diffusivity (MD), which measures the non-directional diffusion of water molecules. Generally, higher FA corresponds to lower MD. Unfortunately, the literature is largely equivocal with regard to these measures; some studies have reported increased FA and decreased MD (Arfanakis et al., 2002; Miles et al., 2008), whereas others have reported decreased FA and increased MD (Bazarian et al., 2007; Mayer et al., 2010) following concussion. Some have argued that FA and MD are dependent on time since injury, with decreased FA and increased MD reported in patients with persistent symptoms or impairment following concussion (Lipton et al., 2008; Niogi et al., 2008). One meta-analysis of DTI findings suggested an overall trend in elevated FA in the acute phase and depressed FA in the chronic phase following concussion (Eierud et al., 2014). Moreover, findings reported in acute and early subacute postinjury phases appear to be even less consistent than those reported from later subacute and chronic time periods. Additionally, the areas of the brain that demonstrate changes in FA and MD following concussion vary (Cubon, Putukian, Boyer, & Dettwiler, 2011).

Recent studies have provided evidence for the utility of DTI in patients in the first few days following concussion (Babcock, Yuan, Leach, Nash, & Wade, 2015). The severity of concussion may also play a role in the utility of DTI findings. For example, Lange and colleagues (2015) reported positive DTI findings that differentiated controls from symptomatic concussed patients but not from asymptomatic concussed patients. Given a publication bias for positive radiologic findings, it is likely that negative studies regarding DTI have been performed but not published. Considering the inconsistent nature of the findings, DTI may not yet be ready for clinical application in the assessment of patients with concussion.

High-Definition Fiber Tracking

High-definition fiber tracking (HDFT) applies mathematical algorithms to conventional DTI findings to examine the integrity of tracts of white matter (Shin et al., 2014). DTI is a type of MRI that allows imaging of the interconnected white matter in the brain. The two most common metrics that are used to assess HDFT findings are *spread*, the density of white matter tracts, and *symmetry*, the degree to which white matter tracts in each brain hemisphere are similar. In short, spread represents the thickness of branches of tracts, and symmetry represents the consistency between tracts on each side of the brain.

We are currently conducting studies at the University of Pittsburgh on HDFT and concussion (see Figure 4.3). We recently concluded a study funded by the Head Health Initiative from General Electric and the National Football League. In our study, we determined whether damage to white matter tracts in adolescents and young adults could be detected in the first 1 to 14 days following concussion and whether damage in white matter tracts corresponded to clinical symptoms and impairment. We also determined whether evidence of repair to white matter tracts on HDFT corresponded to clinical

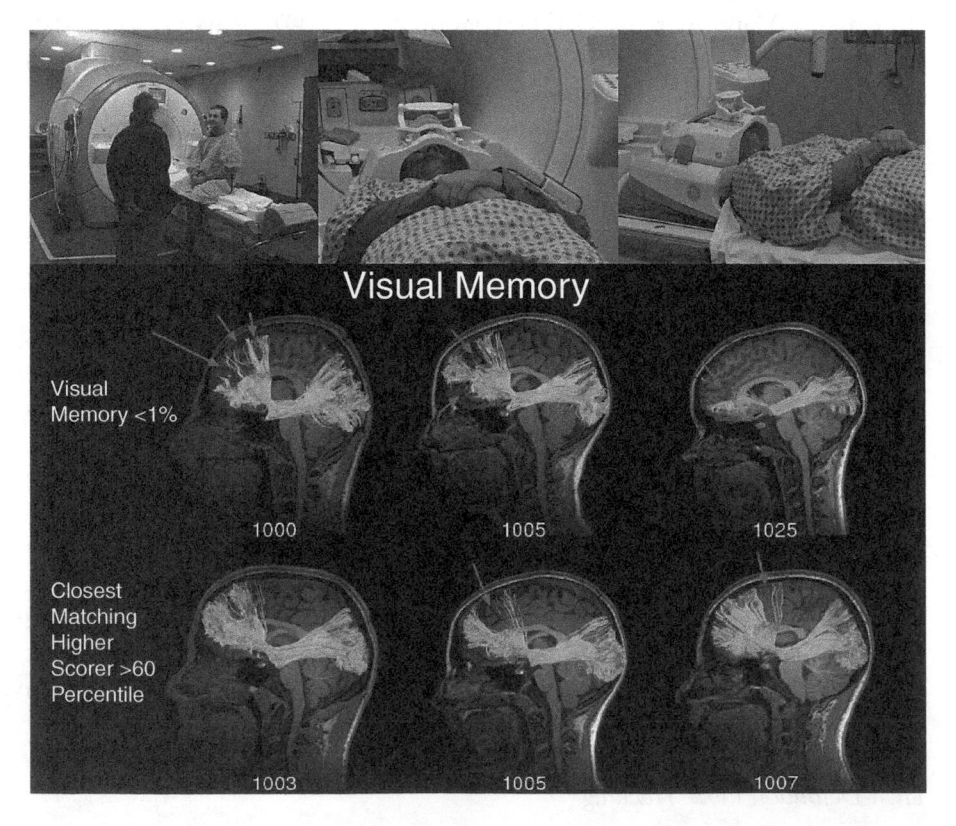

Figure 4.3. High-definition fiber tracking studies at the University of Pittsburgh showing the scanner procedure (top three photos) and comparison of the frontal occipital fasciculus tract of patients with and without visual memory impairment following concussion.

recovery (i.e., date of medical clearance). Our preliminary findings suggest that white damage in certain tracts as measured by HDFT corresponded to clinical findings. Specifically, we found that worse cognitive performance was associated with less spread in tracts such as the cingulum, a region of the limbic system that connects areas of the midbrain and is associated with memory and learning. We also found that improvements in clinical symptoms and impairment were associated with increased spread. This finding is similar to results reported by Presson et al. (2015) in a study of HDFT and neuropsychological outcomes in patients with TBI. Our findings also suggested that HDFT tracts demonstrated greater density or evidence of repair as time from injury increased. This finding brings up an important question: "Does repair to the brain continue even after clinical recovery appears to have occurred?" More research in this area is needed to answer this important question that might have implications for determining safe return to activity for patients following a concussion.

Strengths of HDFT include identification of functional brain tracts that reflect specific functional impairment. As such, HDFT could provide a good assessment of brain recovery following concussion. However, HDFT currently requires the use of human tractographers to interpret damage to specific tracts, which is similar to current approaches to reading and interpreting structural MRI findings. Evolving approaches that use automated analysis of tracts may provide a more objective measure, but additional research is still needed.

Single Photon Emission Computed Tomography/Positron Emission Tomography

Both single photon emission computed tomography (SPECT) and positron emission tomography (PET) assess functional changes in brain metabolism following a concussion; they assess regional blood flow and glucose metabolism in the brain, respectively. Unfortunately, both SPECT and PET are more invasive than other neuroimaging in that an injection of a radioisotope tracer or contrast is required. Therefore, they are not appropriate for children and are currently used only for research purposes. Both approaches have provided compelling evidence of neurometabolic changes in the brain following a concussion (Byrnes et al., 2014). PET imaging is correlated to neuropsychological findings following concussion (Ruff et al., 1994). More recently, PET findings may help identify blast injury in the brain (Mendez et al., 2013) and patients who are malingering versus those with a brain injury (Spadoni, Kosheleva, Buchsbaum, & Simmons, 2015).

Among the strengths of PET/SPECT scans are that they image the metabolic component of concussion and assess both blood flow and metabolism in the brain. Moreover, SPECT is relatively available and inexpensive. Unfortunately, both techniques involve invasive procedures and are time-consuming, and PET is expensive and requires highly specialized equipment that is not widely available.

Magnetic Resonance Spectroscopy Imaging

Similar to PET imaging, magnetic resonance spectroscopy imaging (MRSI) assesses the underlying metabolic changes in the brain associated with concussion. Specifically, MRSI uses high Tesla (7 Tesla) MRIs to measure concentrations of molecular weight particles in the brain. (Tesla refers to the strength of the magnetic field; typical MRIs have 1.5 or 3 Tesla strength.) Typically, MRSI focuses on specific brain regions (e.g., hippocampus) to determine the concentration of a variety of neurometabolic substrates. The commonly measured outcomes in MRSI are choline (Ch), associated with damage to cell membranes; creatine (Cr), related to energy production and regulation; and N-acetyl aspartate (NAA), associated with fluid balance and myelination of neurons. In general, decreased NAA and increased Ch and Cr are associated with injury to the brain (Govindaraju et al., 2004). Often a ratio of NAA/Ch or Cr is used in MRSI, with lower ratios representing evidence of injury to the brain.

Currently, we are conducting research that uses MRSI to differentiate blast mild TBI and posttraumatic stress disorder (PTSD) in military veterans, because these conditions share many clinical symptoms and are often difficult to distinguish. This research follows up on work by de Lanerolle and colleagues (2014) that suggested that MRSI may be useful in detecting the localized neuronal injury following exposure to blast injury. Our preliminary findings suggest that MRSI is useful in delineating patients with only blast mild TBI from those with only PTSD (Kontos, Van Cott, et al., 2017). Specifically, we found that a lower ratio of NAA/Ch in anterior regions of the hippocampus, combined with impaired cognitive performance, may be useful in differentiating these two sets of patients. In addition, both cognitive and vestibular/oculomotor impairments were correlated with decreased NAA/Ch ratios, suggesting that functional impairments correspond to localized injury in the hippocampus following blast injury. Thus, MRSI may be a useful tool to assess metabolic damage associated with blast-related mild TBI. However, more research is needed to determine whether these findings are applicable to nonblast (blunt) brain injuries. To that end, we are currently conducting research with MRSI in civilian and sport populations with blunt concussions.

Overall, MRSI offers an approach that measures metabolic function in specific regions of the brain (some approaches involving whole brain analyses are coming online), can be done in conjunction with structural MRI and DTI (i.e., does not add a lot of additional scan time), can measure deeper structures of the brain like the hippocampus, and does not require injected contrast. MRSI can reliably measure only some of the metabolic compounds in the brain following concussion. Until recently, most high-quality MRSI images required the use of a 7 Tesla MRI, which is costly and available in only a few institutions. However, reliable and detailed images can now be performed at 3 Tesla.

Near-Infrared Spectroscopy

Near-infrared spectroscopy (NIRS) is an optical imaging tool that assesses cerebrovascular blood flow. The NIRS approach was born from the pulse oximeters used to monitor oxygen saturation in patients. Essentially, NIRS and functional NIRS (fNIRS) provide a signal that is analogous to the BOLD signal from fMRI and allows us to monitor cerebrovascular blood flow in the brain. Unlike fMRI, however, fNIRS uses much less expensive equipment (a complete research system currently runs about $75,000–$100,000), is portable, and can even be used while a subject is moving (Huppert, Hoge, Diamond, Franceschini, & Boas, 2006). The fNIRS uses a similar stimulus–response paradigm as fMRI, wherein subjects perform a task while the fNIRS unit simultaneously records cerebrovascular blood flow (see Figure 4.4). The

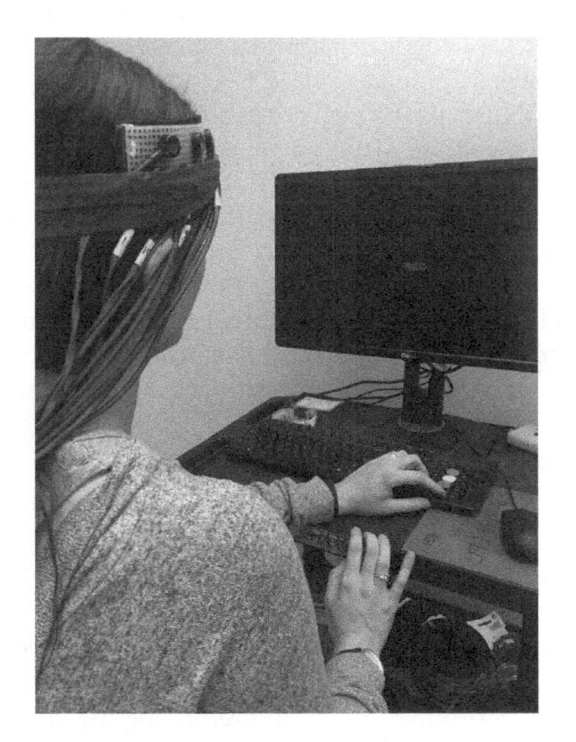

Figure 4.4. Functional near-infrared spectroscopy records blood during a reaction time task.

fNIRS signal is processed using a series of source emitters and detectors that use a light-emitting diode lamp to penetrate to a depth of 8 millimeters in the cortical regions of the brain. The refracted light is then processed and separated into oxygenated and deoxygenated hemoglobin values. This information then allows us to determine the temporal and spatial activity of cerebrovascular blood flow.

Researchers have only recently begun using fNIRS to assess patients with concussion (Kontos, Huppert, et al., 2014). We have an fNIRS system in our Concussion Research Laboratory at the University of Pittsburgh that we are using in several ongoing studies. We have published preliminary findings using fNIRS in patients with concussion (Kontos, Huppert, et al., 2014). We examined fNIRS during the performance of a computerized neurocognitive testing (ImPACT) in a small sample ($N = 14$) of concussed patients and healthy controls. We reported that concussed patients had reduced brain activation during the performance of word, visual and working memory, and symbol match tasks. Specifically, we found reduced activation in the right and left frontal areas of the brain during the performance of cognitive tasks. In addition, the overall behavioral performance (percentage correct and reaction time) in concussed patients corroborated the fNIRS findings. These preliminary findings are promising, and we hope to gain better insight into the utility of fNIRS as an optical imaging tool for concussions from our ongoing research in this area.

In general, fNIRS allows good combined spatial–temporal resolution, is portable, and has the ability to measure brain activity during the performance of tasks and movement, much like fMRI. However, fNIRS has limited ability to penetrate into the cortical areas of the brain beyond a few millimeters (< 10 mm) and is, therefore, unable to assess deeper brain structures. The fNIRS imaging process is prone to a high noise-to-signal ratio from the optical signal, which can obfuscate subtle findings. Finally, because fNIRS is an indirect measure conducted through the hair, scalp, and skull, there is greater potential for measurement error from these confounding structures.

Electroencephalography and Brain Network Activation

Since the 1950s and 1960s, researchers have used electrophysiological measures, including EEG and quantitative EEG (qEEG), to measure the effects of concussion in the human brain (Hiddema, 1963). An EEG indirectly measures electrical brain activity in cortical regions through a series of electrodes on the scalp. A variety of different electrical waves are measured, including alpha, beta, theta, and delta waves. The qEEG approach utilizes a computer and algorithms to assist in interpreting the visual findings from EEG. Both EEG and qEEG have been used to identify concussion acutely (McCrea, Prichep, Powell, Chabot, & Barr, 2010) and to monitor subacute and longer term effects of concussion in the brain (Slobounov, Sebastianelli, & Hallett, 2012). Recently, researchers have even begun combining EEG with exertion protocols to assess readiness for return to play with tentative support for this approach (Gay et al., 2015). Researchers have reported that EEG abnormalities may persist up to 30 days postinjury, even in patients who make a clinical recovery (Cao, Tutwiler, & Slobounov, 2008).

Another approach to EEG involves the application of evoked response potentials (ERP), which represent the electrical activity that occurs in response to a stimulus. Typically, researchers measure the latency, amplitude, and frequency of EEG waves during ERPs. However, a new approach called brain network activation (BNA) uses an algorithm to identify functional network dynamics and quantify a concussed individual's network activity to that of a healthy normative or reference group (Kontos, Reches, et al., 2016). In short, BNA allows us to map temporal–spatial EEG/ERP activity to provide a visual representation of the functional connectivity in the brain following concussion (see Figure 4.5).

We recently conducted a 2-year study of BNA in concussed and healthy matched controls at 1-week intervals over 1 month. Our preliminary findings suggest that BNA is good at differentiating concussed individuals from controls and is useful in tracking recovery following concussion. In addition, BNA was correlated with clinical assessments, including symptoms and cognitive impairment. Initial findings also indicate that BNA may be able to help differentiate among concussion clinical profiles. For example, in a recent study of high school–aged and young adult athletes with concussion, we reported that BNA was useful in differentiating patients with posttraumatic migraine following concussion from those without migraine and healthy matched controls (Kontos, Reches, et al., 2016).

Although more research on BNA is needed, the initial results are promising. However, reported findings suggest that a single BNA score may not be sufficient across all types of concussion (Eckner et al., 2016). Overall, EEG/ ERP offers good temporal resolution and has a relatively low cost compared with other neuroimaging approaches, but provides limited spatial resolution relative to other methods (e.g., MRI/DTI) and takes considerable time to set up to obtain a good initial signal. Like fNIRS, EEG/ERP approaches are susceptible to noise from the electrical signals traveling through hair, scalp, and skull.

Magnetoencephalography

Magnetoencephalography (MEG) involves the measurement of magnetic fields or wave currents that reflect neuronal activity in gray matter of the brain during the performance of a task or at resting state, much like fMRI (Lee & Huang, 2014). Preliminary findings suggest that MEG can

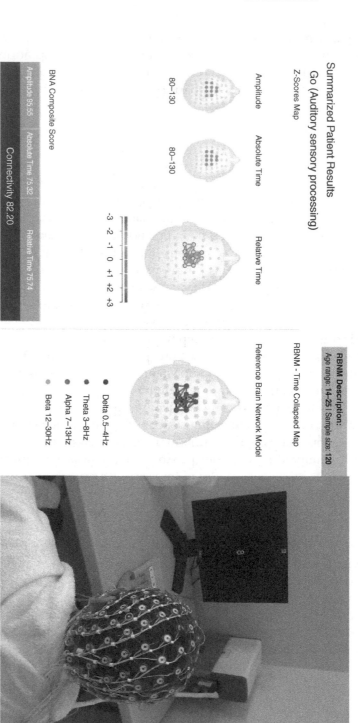

Summarized Patient Results

Go (Auditory sensory processing)

Z-Scores Map

RBNM Description:
Age range: **14-25** | Sample size: **120**

| Amplitude | Absolute Time | Relative Time | Reference Brain Network Model |

80–130   80–130

-3 -2 -1 0 +1 +2 +3

RBNM - Time Collapsed Map

● Delta 0.5–4Hz
● Theta 3–8Hz
● Alpha 7–13Hz
● Beta 12–30Hz

BNA Composite Score

Amplitude 95.55	Absolute Time 75.32	Relative Time 75.74
Connectivity 82.20		

Figure 4.5. Brain network activation maps brain connectivity (left image) using EEG/evoked response potential data captured during the performance of a task (right image). RBNM = reference brain network model; BNA = brain network activation.

detect the presence of abnormal slow wave (i.e., delta waves) activity in the brain (Lewine et al., 2007). These abnormal brain waves appear to represent structural damage to the brain and have been correlated to DTI findings (M. X. Huang et al., 2009). Researchers have used MEG to accurately identify abnormal delta wave patterns in 77% of patients with blunt mild TBI (M. X. Huang, Nichols, et al., 2012). Research has also supported correlations between MEG findings and cognitive impairment following concussion (Swan et al., 2015). Unfortunately, very few MEG units are available outside of large academic institutions, and most are focused on research applications only. As a result, the use of MEG with patients following concussion is limited to a handful of studies.

Blood Biomarkers

No accepted or approved clinical blood biomarker test for concussion is available. Although several companies and researchers have made claims to the contrary, to date, no single blood biomarker is effective in detecting concussion (diagnosis) or measuring recovery (prognosis). In short, there is no "blood test" for concussion. On the other hand, few singular blood tests for complicated medical diagnoses or conditions (e.g., obesity, psychiatric disorders, heart disease) exist. In fact, the more we learn about these conditions, the more we appreciate how complex they are; it is unlikely that a single blood biomarker can accurately identify disease or injury and its resolution.

The term *biomarker* is often applied to any biological or physiological indicator of disease or injury. Typically, evidence of the biomarker, which reflects change in some biomolecule (e.g., protein, metabolite, neurotransmitter), is derived from blood or other body fluids such as cerebral spinal fluid (CSF), urine, saliva, or sweat. In the case of concussion, CSF would provide the most ideal source for a biomarker because of its direct relation to damage in the brain. Unfortunately, acquiring CSF is invasive, and the risks far outweigh any potential benefits for patients with concussion. Consequently, the most common source for concussion biomarkers is peripheral blood, which represents an indirect assessment of the concentration of any biomolecule in the brain following concussion. The use of peripheral blood also presents challenges related to the use of venipuncture, which is viewed as invasive for a mild injury such as concussion and is not as tolerable as a finger stick.

Additionally, many of the blood biomarkers denigrate quickly following concussion, thereby requiring early (i.e., within 24–48 hours of injury) assessment (Papa et al., 2016). Although this approach is potentially useful in diagnosing concussions in the acute phase, most patients, aside from those presenting to an emergency department, are not examined by clinicians within this time period. For the same reason, testing for specific blood biomarkers is not useful for these patients; the relevant biomarkers are no longer present in the bloodstream after 48 hours of a concussion.

Conceptually, blood biomarkers may offer a more objective and potentially rapid assessment of concussion and its effects than current clinical assessments. This premise is based on the concept that all concussions share some consistent primary injury features associated with the injury, including damage to cerebrovascular and neuronal structures (Dash, Zhao, Hergenroeder, & Moore, 2010). Using this framework, it is reasonable that concussions might produce a biomarker distinguishable from other neuroinflammatory and related diseases or injuries. However, the symptoms, impairments, and other functional and concomitant structural damages, which are collectively referred to as *secondary injury from concussion*, are heterogeneous and inconsistent (Dash et al., 2010). As a result, and because of the heterogeneity of concussion, it is unlikely that any single blood biomarker test will be accurate across all patients with concussions.

However, the heterogeneity of concussion does not imply that blood biomarkers have no role in its assessment. To the contrary, blood biomarkers may provide more objective evidence to support functional assessments of the various concussion clinical profiles, inform prognosis, and monitor recovery and the effectiveness of clinical treatments. Glial fibrillary acidic protein (GFAP; Papa et al., 2014) and ubiquitin C-terminal hydrolase-L1 (UCH-L1) may hold promise as potential biomarkers for concussion (Papa et al., 2016). However, UCH-L1 findings are less robust than those for GFAP in children (Rhine, Babcock, Zhang, Leach, & Wade, 2016). In addition, time of testing may affect the effectiveness of blood biomarkers; GFAP can be detected up to 7 days postinjury, whereas UCH-L1 may only be evident in the first 24 hours following injury (Papa et al., 2016). Additional large-scale studies focusing on blood biomarkers for specific clinical profiles of concussion are warranted. An overview of the emerging blood biomarkers for detecting and assessing recovery following concussion is provided in Table 4.1.

Although single blood biomarkers are not available, it is likely that a combination of different blood biomarkers may provide a more useful approach. A panel or assay of blood biomarkers in different combinations and levels may be the most useful approach. Similar approaches have been used in other complex diseases such as heart disease and certain types of cancer. Using this assay approach, researchers may identify a series of blood biomarkers that, when viewed in combination and in varying levels, represent different clinical profiles for concussion. This approach is reflective of the heterogeneous nature of concussion; it may inform early identification of concussion profiles that inform earlier intervention and potentially provide a marker for improvement following intervention (Wang et al., 2005).

TABLE 4.1
Overview of Emerging Blood Biomarkers for Concussion

Biomarker	Description	Indication
S100B	A calcium-binding protein in astrocytes that regulates intracellular calcium; however, it may be nonspecific to brain injury.	Marker of severity and postconcussion symptoms.
Glial fibrillary acidic protein	A glial specific neuroinflammatory marker.	Acute marker of brain injury.
Neuron-specific enolase	An isozyme related to neuronal injury.	Marker for severity of brain injury.
Tau	A protein that accumulates into bundles and includes phosphorylated tau (*P-tau*), cleaved tau (*C-tau*), and total tau protein; it measures axonal disruption.	Total *tau* protein is a marker for severity and poor outcome.
Ubiquitin C-terminal hydrolase L1	A protein related to neuronal injury.	Acute marker for brain injury (< 1 hour); marker for injury severity.

SAMPLE COMPREHENSIVE APPROACH
TO ASSESSING CONCUSSION

Any comprehensive approach to assessing concussion should be informed by the underlying conceptual approach and take available resources into consideration. For example, exertion-based testing may be difficult to implement in a small clinic/office setting staffed by a single clinician. However, at a minimum, a comprehensive approach to assessing concussion should include the following components: (a) clinical exam and interview, (b) symptoms, (c) neurocognitive assessment, (d) vestibular and oculomotor screening, and (e) exertion-based testing. In this section we describe each of these components as assessed in our clinic.

The clinical exam and interview component includes a complete medical and injury history, psychosocial history, and exam focused on injury characteristics and risk factors. We assess symptoms using a combination of self-report questionnaires including the Post-Concussion Symptom Scale administered at the beginning and end of neurocognitive testing and again after we complete exertion-based testing (if applicable) and open-ended assessments of symptoms during the clinical interview. For children and adolescents, we also ask parents or legal guardians about the patient symptoms and behavior changes.

The neurocognitive test (ImPACT) is completed on the computer and includes tests of visual and verbal memory, reaction time, and processing speed. Ideally, baseline measures of cognitive performance are available; if they are not, we use normative data for similar age and gender groups. We use the VOMS to screen for vestibular and oculomotor symptoms and impairment. Our exertion-based testing protocol consists of both dynamic and aerobic-based physical exertion components, followed by symptom assessments. Exertion-based protocols may not be indicated during the initial clinical visit if a patient is grossly symptomatic or impaired. Therefore, the use of exertion-based protocols is predicated on the tolerance level of the individual patient. However, we find that many patients experience an increase in symptoms following dynamic exertion that involves lateral whole-body and head movements but not after aerobic exertion.

Although the timing of the administration of the approach discussed here may vary depending on resources and patient flow, we generally use the following sequence: (a) symptoms and neurocognitive assessment, (b) clinical interview and exam, (c) vestibular and oculomotor screening, and (d) exertion-based testing. The order of testing is also determined by whether symptoms worsen during the process or remain stable. Therefore, at the initial appointment symptoms should be assessed following different components of the evaluation that may exacerbate symptoms and at different time points during the clinical interview. A general worsening of symptoms may be indicative of a cognitive/fatigue clinical profile, whereas provocation of symptoms following specific tests, such as vestibular screening, may reflect a vestibular or other clinical profile.

CONCLUSION

No single assessment is available to reliably identify and track recovery following concussion. A comprehensive approach to assessing concussion involving multiple domains is needed. Brief acute, or in the case of sport, on-field measures of concussion are useful to identify suspected injuries. A comprehensive clinical assessment begins with a thorough medical, psychosocial, and injury history and in-depth clinical exam and interview. Additional assessments of cognitive, neuromotor, vestibular, oculomotor/vision, and psychological domains are also indicated. Several promising techniques for assessing concussion involving neuroimaging and blood biomarkers have emerged in recent years. However, most of these approaches (fMRI, PET) are time-consuming and involve expensive specialized equipment and personnel. Initial evidence suggests that some less expensive approaches, including fNIRS and BNA, have the potential to complement current behavioral concussion assessments, but more research is warranted. Overall, the key to assessing patients with a concussion is to use a comprehensive approach that covers multiple domains (symptoms, cognitive, neuromotor, and psychological) and employs a variety of techniques (history, exam, interview, questionnaires, and computerized testing).

5

TARGETED TREATMENT STRATEGIES FOR CONCUSSION

Concussion is treatable. On the surface this seems to be a simple and straightforward declarative statement. However, the notion that concussion is actually treatable (as opposed to manageable) is nothing short of a seismic shift in the approach to clinical care for patients with concussion. In a 2015 Harris Poll of 2,000 adults in the United States, more than 70% did not realize that concussions are treatable. More important, the statement about concussion being treatable versus manageable connotes that treatment for concussion may go beyond passive "wait and see" approaches to include more active and progressive approaches. Concussion treatment is in its infancy, but we believe that the field needs to shift from management-based approaches to more active and targeted approaches that draw on clinical profiles to provide patients with the best clinical outcomes. As such, we advocate for a targeted approach to treating concussion that is progressive, interdisciplinary, and focused on the clinical profiles-based findings from the assessments described in Chapter 4.

http://dx.doi.org/10.1037/0000087-006
Concussion: A Clinical Profile Approach to Assessment and Treatment, by A. P. Kontos and M. W. Collins
Copyright © 2018 by the American Psychological Association. All rights reserved.

FRAMEWORK FOR TARGETED APPROACHES TO TREATING CONCUSSION: A PROGRESSIVE APPROACH

In Chapter 1 we introduced concussion clinical profiles, which provide clinicians with a pseudotaxonomic system for conceptualizing concussion and its various manifestations. The underlying notion behind the use of clinical profiles for concussion is to allow for more targeted, efficient, and effective treatment strategies to match each profile. Clinical profiles are identified using the comprehensive assessment approach outlined in Chapter 4. After a patient's clinical profiles have been determined, the next challenge is to decide which profile requires immediate treatment. In other words, we need to triage the clinical profiles to deal with the profile that is most problematic or pressing first, rather than adopt a blanket approach that treats everything simultaneously. The triage approach will allow for the most substantial initial improvement, which can set the stage for a more rapid recovery. Otherwise, we run the risk of "digging a lot of shallow wells" without much positive effect for the patient. Instead, we want to "dig a deep well" that allows the greatest initial impact on the patient's symptoms and impairment. A targeted approach to treating concussion clinical profiles should be progressive using primary, secondary, and tertiary categories to prioritize treatment (see Figure 1.3).

After the primary concussion clinical profile is identified, a targeted and active treatment plan to address that profile should be initiated. However, it is unlikely that a single clinician can effectively provide treatment for all clinical profiles. It is our belief that it takes a "village" of clinical experts from a variety of disciplines to effectively treat concussion. To implement such an approach, clinicians should have access to an interdisciplinary team that encompasses multiple areas of expertise to provide well-rounded and effective care.

THE INTERDISCIPLINARY CONCUSSION TEAM

The best approach for treating concussion involves an interdisciplinary clinical team representing multiple specialties that is coordinated by a clinician who acts as a central hub for coordinating patient care and has specialty training in concussion care (see Figure 1.4). This approach is similar to the role of a "point guard" on a basketball team—the player who makes sure that the right people get the ball at the right time to maximize the effectiveness of the team. No single specialty has a monopoly on being the coordinating clinician. A clinical neuropsychologist; neurologist; sports medicine, physical medicine and rehabilitation physician; or other clinician could assume this role.

Regardless of who is in this position, the coordinating clinician needs to have a strong referral provider network to address the various treatment foci discussed in the subsequent sections of this chapter. Among the providers that should be included in the interdisciplinary team are vestibular and physical therapists, neuro-optometrists, neurologists, neurosurgeons, psychologists, radiologists, and athletic trainers. To facilitate patients into appropriate care, strong referral networks need to be maintained by clinicians who typically provide the initial care to patients with concussion. Among the common initial care providers for this injury are emergency physicians, athletic trainers, general practitioners, and family and pediatric physicians.

We realize that many clinicians do not have access to an interdisciplinary team of providers to assess and treat a patient with a concussion. Some clinicians may be located in rural areas and have limited access to clinicians from other specialties. For example, one of the authors (Anthony Kontos) directed the North Coast Sports Concussion Program at Humboldt State University in Northern California (about 1.5 hours south of Oregon on the Redwood Coast). In Humboldt, access to providers was limited, particularly for patients living in the coastal mountain range and those on American Indian tribal lands. Further complicating matters at schools was that the state of California did not recognize certified athletic trainers. As a result, the only option for concussion assessment and treatment at these schools was often an emergency medical technician or school nurse with limited or no training in concussion care.

Recently we worked with the U.S. Department of Defense on a project called TEAM TBI, which brings military personnel with chronic concussion symptoms from around the United States to the University of Pittsburgh Medical Center for a multiday comprehensive assessment and targeted treatments. We found that many military personnel return to their base or home (if they are veterans) where they have limited access to appropriate clinicians. As a result of these barriers to an interdisciplinary team for treating concussion, several approaches have begun to be developed to allow for better access to an interdisciplinary team approach. One method being explored is the use of telemedicine. A colleague of ours, R. J. Elbin at the University of Arkansas, is working on a telemedicine program for concussion to provide better access to care among rural patients in Arkansas. Another strategy involves the use of tablet- and smartphone-based applications in conjunction with activity monitoring devices that allow patients to engage in rehabilitation remotely under the supervision of clinicians. Although these approaches may enhance clinicians' ability to incorporate an interdisciplinary approach with their patients, they are not yet ready for prime time. However, within the next decade or so, we are likely to have access to both telemedicine and remote monitoring approaches to enhance patient care for concussion.

One final note regarding interdisciplinary care for concussion pertains to health care coverage and reimbursement. Many current health care insurance programs offer some coverage for the initial assessment and evaluation for a concussion. However, access to specialized treatment providers, such as vestibular and vision therapists, may be limited or not covered at all in current plans. As a result, many patients cannot afford the care that has been prescribed to them. Clinicians from psychology, neurology, physical therapy, and other fields should lobby collectively for coverage for specialized treatment of concussion. Otherwise, the level of care for patients will continue to be limited by a lack of coverage for the care they need, ultimately resulting in greater health care costs for related chronic problems down the road.

REST AND ACCOMMODATIVE STRATEGIES
AFTER CONCUSSION

Prescribed Rest

Prescribed rest is an intuitive and widely embraced therapy for many medical conditions. The theory for prescribed rest is as follows: After a concussion, metabolic demand increases and adenosine triphosphate (ATP) reserves are limited; cognitive and physical activity may require oxygen and ATP from recovering neurons. Prescribed rest includes restriction of a variety of both physical (e.g., aerobic exercise, resistance training, dynamic movements) and cognitive (e.g., schoolwork, reading, computer work) activities. The purpose of prescribed rest is twofold: (a) to protect the patient from subsequent injury to the brain during the vulnerable acute time period following a concussion (Schnadower, Vazquez, Lee, Dayan, & Roskind, 2007), and (b) to provide down time for the brain to heal while avoiding exacerbation of symptoms and impairment from the added load of physical and cognitive activity (Giza, Griesbach, & Hovda, 2005; Griesbach, Hovda, Molteni, Wu, & Gomez-Pinilla, 2004).

Restricting exposure to another injury to the brain during the vulnerable acute time period is critical (especially to prevent second impact syndrome), and that can be accomplished through restriction of contact (e.g., tackling in American football, checking in ice hockey) and "at risk" physical activities (e.g., working on a ladder, running an obstacle course in the military). Other physical activities such as walking, running, and noncontact training carry negligible risk for a second injury to the brain. As such, the restriction of these activities is driven largely by the second purpose for prescribed rest, allowing the brain time to heal. Regardless of the underlying theory, additional research is needed to better understand the dose and timing of prescribed rest.

Should we advise patients to rest only in the acute phase postinjury? Should patients with chronic concussion symptoms be advised to rest? Should we prescribe cognitive and physical rest together, or should we use each only in certain situations with certain patients? All of these questions have yet to be addressed empirically and warrant further inquiry to better inform the use of prescribed rest in patients following concussion.

Conceptually, prescribed physical and cognitive rest is an intervention for concussion, albeit an inactive one. In fact, prescribed rest is the most common strategy used for patients with concussion (Broglio et al., 2014; Giza et al., 2013; P. McCrory et al., 2013). A recent Harris Poll (2015) indicated that among the 33% of patients receiving some form of treatment for concussion, more than half (51%) were prescribed some form of rest as the only treatment. However, as the 2013 Institute of Medicine and National Research Council report on concussion in sport stated, "there is little evidence regarding the efficacy of rest following concussion or to inform the best timing and approach for return to activity. . . ."; the report recommends that "randomized controlled trials" (RCTs) be conducted "to determine the efficacy of physical or cognitive rest . . ." We fully agree. What we do know about the effectiveness of prescribed rest following concussion comes largely from expert consensus (e.g., Broglio et al., 2014; Giza et al., 2013; P. McCrory et al., 2013) and a handful of studies (e.g., N. J. Brown et al., 2014; Moser, Glatts, & Schatz, 2012) that focused on patients from sports medicine clinics and thereby is limited in scope.

Moser and colleagues (2012) reported that prescribed physical rest was effective in reducing recovery time in symptomatic patients seen a few weeks following their concussion. Similarly, in a study looking at cognitive rest and activity, N. J. Brown and colleagues (2014) reported that patients who engaged in more cognitive activity (i.e., less cognitive rest) took longer to recover and reported more symptoms. Both studies provided some of the first empirical data to examine the effectiveness of rest following concussion, but they were limited by nonrandomized assignment of rest and included only a selective population of patients who sought specialty care for their concussion. Consequently, these patients may have been more likely to have greater symptoms and impairment than other patients. We speculate that patients such as these, who have a more organic burden (i.e., severity) following concussion, may benefit more from prescribed rest, whereas other patients with less severe injury may benefit more from earlier active interventions. Certain signs such as loss of consciousness, amnesia, and confusion/disorientation may reflect the severity of neurometabolic dysfunction following a concussion (Craton & Leslie, 2014). These signs may also indicate hemodynamic, structural, and electrical alterations related to unmet metabolic demands (Wells, Goodkin, & Griesbach, 2016).

Preclinical research supports the notion that the stress of physical (Griesbach, Hovda, et al., 2004) and cognitive (Reger et al., 2012) activity following concussion is contraindicated for neuroplasticity, neuroinflammation, and cognitive function. Although we do not fully understand the mechanism for these effects, it is thought to be related to increased demand for energy in the brain at a time when it is metabolically compromised (Giza & Hovda, 2014), together with a hyperresponsiveness (through increased glucocorticoid) to stress from activity (Grønli et al., 2006; Schaaf, de Jong, de Kloet, & Vreugdenhil, 1998). As such, patients presenting with signs of concussion may benefit from avoiding further disruption of cellular function and cerebral metabolism and stress from physical and cognitive activity. What is less clear is whether a concussion that elicits only symptoms (particularly those that are less concussion-specific, such as anxiety and mood-related symptoms) reflects a similar neurometabolic injury (Cassidy et al., 2014). One component of treatment that often accompanies prescribed rest and facilitates a reduction in activity is *accommodation*, or the adjustment of one's environment and functioning to avoid exacerbating symptoms and impairment, while maintaining some level of preinjury performance or function.

Prescribed rest is typically viewed as an innocuous treatment recommendation (i.e., one that carries with it limited negative consequences). Therefore, clinicians may believe that by prescribing rest they are doing no harm to their patients. In most cases this belief is accurate. However, research shows that prescribed rest, particularly prolonged rest, may actually exacerbate symptoms through several mechanisms. A review of research on bed rest, long considered "intuitive" for recovery of many medical conditions, showed bed rest to be ineffective in all conditions studied (Allen, Glasziou, & Del Mar, 1999). The only published randomized clinical study of bed rest for treatment of concussion, comparing no bed rest and 6 days of bed rest in 107 adults, showed no benefit to rest (de Kruijk, Leffers, Meerhoff, Rutten, & Twijnstra, 2002). Research on rest for conditions other than concussion suggests that rest may cause patients to dwell on their symptoms (i.e., hypervigilance), become socially isolated, and disrupt their normal routines (Cacioppo, Hawkley, Norman, & Berntson, 2011; Colloca & Finniss, 2012; Ponsford et al., 2012). Prescribed rest sets up a negative expectation for recovery; some might interpret it to mean that "your concussion is so bad that we need to shut everything down," which may in and of itself lead to a prolonged recovery. In support of this notion, Zuckerbraun and colleagues recently reported that just providing instructions for prescribed rest following a concussion was associated with higher symptom reports (Zuckerbraun, Atabaki, Collins, Thomas, & Gioia, 2014).

We believe that certain types of patients (e.g., somaticizers) are more likely than other patients to experience these negative outcomes following prescribed rest. Findings from our recent study bear this out: Somatic patients reported higher symptoms several weeks following their concussion than other patients (Root et al., 2016). Specific to concussion, D. G. Thomas, Apps, Hoffmann, McCrea, and Hammeke (2015) reported that among patients in the emergency department who were randomized to early, prolonged prescribed physical and cognitive rest reported more postconcussive symptoms. Of note, these patients reported more emotional symptoms throughout recovery, which may be a result of the hypervigilance and social isolation mechanisms mentioned earlier.

Previously, Majerske and colleagues (2008) reported that patients with low levels of physical and cognitive activity in the first month following concussion experienced more negative outcomes than those who were moderately active. These researchers also found high levels of activity in the first month following concussion to be deleterious to patients. These findings bring to the discussion the role of time since injury, which may also influence the effectiveness of prescribed rest. It is generally accepted that use of earlier rest is most effective following concussion, with diminishing returns thereafter. However, it is less clear whether the use of rest later in the recovery process is effective and if so, how long postinjury does it remain effective.

Researchers have intimated that patients with chronic concussive symptoms may in fact benefit from more active rehabilitation (e.g., low-level physical activity; P. McCrory et al., 2013), but additional empirical data to support this contention are needed. Overall, for some patients, prescribed physical and cognitive rest may worsen symptoms and impairment and extend recovery. Specifically, a combination of prescribed rest, saturated media coverage of concussion and its effects, and legislation mandating clearance from a health care provider may create a climate that encourages a self-fulfilling prophesy of delayed recovery and prolonged symptoms. Therefore, alternative approaches are warranted. We are learning that more active approaches to treating concussion may enhance recovery for many patients. These patients may benefit from a more active approach that involves earlier prescribed activity.

Accommodations

Similar to prescribed rest, accommodative strategies are designed to minimize the load on patients who have sustained a concussion because they may be susceptible to adverse effects and decreased performance at that time (Ransom et al., 2015). The logic behind accommodative strategies is that targeted, progressive approaches involving appropriate supports may mitigate adverse effects on academic, work, and military performance; integrate patients back into their normal daily routines; and decrease exposure to adverse stimuli and activities that may lengthen recovery time. Any approach to accommodation following a concussion should be targeted to the individual and involve accommodations that match impairment and symptoms per identified clinical profiles. As an example, a patient with a primary vestibular clinical profile may require accommodations at work or school that involve a reduction in busy environments involving a lot of people, movement, and stimuli. Similarly, a patient with a cognitive-fatigue clinical profile may benefit from a greater workload in the earlier part of the day, with increasing accommodations as the day goes on to minimize fatigue and symptoms. Patients with oculomotor clinical profiles may require a reduction in all activities that involve visual input such as tests, reading, or working on a computer until their symptoms resolve or are tolerable.

Blanket accommodations used for all patients may result in worsening of symptoms and impairment and prolonged absence from work, school, sport or military duty. In addition, some patients (and their parents, in the case of school-aged children) may take advantage of accommodations for academic benefit. Other adult-aged patients may exploit accommodations to avoid work activities and prolong worker's compensation or other benefits associated with a delayed return to activities. In our experience, only a small minority of patients use this maladaptive approach. However, the patients who tend to take advantage of accommodations are those with anxiety/mood clinical profiles (or helicopter parents).

For accommodative strategies to be effective, a strong and knowledgeable support system must be in place. Such a system ideally involves family; health care workers; and work, school, and military personnel to maximize the success of these strategies and to provide information regarding the progress of the patient toward a return to normal functioning. Researchers have advocated a progressive, monitored approach to accommodations that promotes gradual return to normal activity without restrictions (Gioia, Glang, Hooper, & Brown, 2016). Specific programs to help guide accommodative strategies should focus first on education and then on the development and implementation of a specific, individualized plan to address symptoms and impairment specific to the patient's clinical profile(s). Several such approaches have been proposed by researchers and clinicians (see Eagan Brown & Vaccaro, 2014; Glang et al., 2015; McAvoy, 2009).

These education/plan-based programs that use an individualized approach enhance outcomes related to accommodations. Specifically, researchers reported significant increases in knowledge of concussion and academic accommodations, as well as successful execution of the plans themselves (Glang et al., 2015). Most plans and research to date have focused on academic accommodations, with little emphasis on work or military duty accommodations aside from the ACE Care Plan–Work accommodations (Gioia & Collins, 2006). Therefore, additional research on accommodative strategies that target a range of vocational and other functional activities across different age groups is warranted. Prolonged accommodations are not indicated as they may result in social isolation and loss of routine that can in turn lead to anxiety, mood disturbance, and withdrawal from other activities.

ACTIVE THERAPIES FOLLOWING CONCUSSION

The idea for active approaches to treating concussion is not new. However, much of the theory for its use is based on research on traumatic brain injury (TBI). Research involving animal studies has demonstrated that an "enriched environment" of physical and cognitive stimulation enhances histologic, cognitive, and behavioral recovery from TBI (e.g., Kovesdi et al., 2011). Preclinical studies document a range of beneficial effects from enriched environments, including decreased lesion size, enhanced dendritic branching, increased trophic factors, and proliferation of progenitor cells (Nithianantharajah & Hannan, 2006). In patients with TBI, cognitive, physical, and social activity has been associated with improved outcome and sparing of hippocampal atrophy (Miller, Colella, Mikulis, Maller, & Green, 2013). Active therapies following a concussion provide an enriched environment for patients—physical activity, social integration, and intellectual stimulation. Moreover, active targeted therapies also may help to rehabituate the systems affected following concussion. For example, active vestibular exercises may promote restoration of vestibular function for a patient with this clinical profile following a concussion. In contrast, a patient with this same clinical profile who is told to rest may not see improvement in vestibular function. In summary, we believe that the use of prescribed rest across all patients and clinical profiles may set the stage for a pattern of behavior (i.e., "sick role") that is likely to continue into the subacute phase when enrichment may be more beneficial. Active strategies may be better than prescribed rest, particularly in the face of persistent symptoms.

The key with any prescribed activity is finding a balance between exposure and recovery such that the patient's symptoms and impairment do not worsen. It is unlikely that prescribed low-level physical and cognitive activities will worsen injury to the brain following a concussion, even though they may temporarily increase symptoms in some patients. At our University of Pittsburgh Medical Center (UPMC) Sports Medicine Concussion Program clinics in Pittsburgh, we have used expose-recover, active approaches to treating concussion for nearly a decade. Among the active approaches that we have found to be useful in treating patients are exertion (i.e., dynamic and aerobic physical activity), vestibular, and vision/oculomotor-based therapies.

Exertion-Based Therapies

There is limited empirical evidence for the effectiveness of exertion-based therapies for patients with concussion. Most of that evidence has centered on patients with chronic postconcussion symptoms. In a small study of 12 patients with chronic symptoms following concussion, Leddy and colleagues (2010) reported that treadmill-based aerobic exercise was effective in reducing symptoms. However, the control group in this study received no treatment, and the treatment was not randomly assigned. In addition, this approach focused only on aerobic exertion, which may not be appropriate for all patients. A recent small randomized clinical trial by Maerlender, Rieman, Lichtenstein, and Condiracci (2015) indicated that low to moderate exertion therapy immediately following concussion did not adversely affect recovery time. However, these researchers reported that high levels of physical exertion were associated with negative effects. These findings echo the results from Majerske et al. (2008) and lend further support for the use of low- to moderate-level exertion following concussion.

One of the challenges to using exertion-based therapies following concussion is the individual variability in the fitness level of patients. Additionally, following a concussion, typical rest-based approaches may result in lost fitness and lower tolerance for physical exertion. Researchers have recently suggested that heart rate variability following concussion is evident even in asymptomatic patients during exertion (Abaji, Curnier, Moore, & Ellemberg, 2016). We previously reported that aerobic fitness variability may affect concussion outcomes (Kontos, Elbin, & Collins, 2006). It is intuitive to postulate that a similar effect would occur in patients with decreased fitness levels following concussion. In fact, Leddy et al. (2010) indicated that athletes (who presumably were more fit than nonathletes) recovered faster from chronic concussion symptoms following exertion than did nonathletes.

In our clinic at UPMC in Pittsburgh, we use combined dynamic and aerobic exertion protocols that are tailored to each patient's clinical profiles and that meet the specific environmental demands of each patient. For example, a patient with a cognitive-fatigue profile may benefit more from aerobic exertion, whereas a patient with vestibular or oculomotor clinical profiles may benefit more from progressive dynamic exertion. Similarly, with regard to environment, a patient who plays ice hockey will need to be able to function in that environment. Therefore, a focus on more anaerobic and lateral dynamic exertion is more appropriate for that patient than it is for a patient who is returning to road cycling or a desk job. Our current approach to exertion-based therapies following concussion is highly individualized and may involve many permutations.

Although we have had great anecdotal success with this approach, it does not lend itself well to research to detect group differences. Therefore, many questions remain regarding the timing, frequency, duration, and intensity of exertion for use with patients following concussion. Researchers and clinicians should work together to answers these questions and to determine which types of exertion are most beneficial to patients with which clinical profiles. Only then will we be able to have a more systematic yet individualized approach to applying exertion-based therapies for patients with specific clinical profiles.

Vestibular Therapies

In our experience, most vestibular dysfunction and symptoms in patients with vestibular clinical profiles following concussion result from disruption in the central vestibular pathways and structures. In brief, centrally mediated vestibular function is adversely affected following concussion, resulting in disequilibrium, imbalance, dizziness, vertigo, and other symptoms and dysfunction (Furman, Raz, & Whitney, 2010). Peripheral vestibular dysfunction appears to be less common following concussion, although prevalence rates are not established in the literature. (For a thorough review of additional vestibular dysfunction following concussion and associated therapies, including those targeting peripheral vestibular issues, see Broglio, Collins, Williams, Mucha, & Kontos, 2015, and Kontos & Ortega, 2011.) These vestibular symptoms and dysfunction are categorized as either vestibulospinal (involving the balance and gait) or vestibulo-ocular (involving integration of visual and vestibular input with the movement of the head and body). The underlying categorization and concomitant symptoms and dysfunction will drive which therapies will be most effective for each patient.

A growing body of evidence suggests that vestibular therapies can help to alleviate vestibular-related symptoms and impairment following a concussion. In fact, in a study of 114 patients both dizziness and imbalance were decreased following vestibular rehabilitation (Alsalaheen et al., 2010). These same researchers reported that these positive effects were obtained after only a single session of vestibular rehabilitation in both adult and adolescent patients. In addition, patients in the same study who completed vestibular rehabilitation exercises also reported being more confident in their ability to maintain balance following injury. However, this study was retrospective in nature and did not include a control group for comparison.

K. J. Schneider and colleagues (2014) extended this initial work by conducting an RCT of the effectiveness of vestibular rehabilitation with 31 adolescent and young adult patients with a concussion. They reported that the patients randomized to the vestibular rehabilitation intervention were nearly 4 times more likely to be recovered by 8 weeks than the control group. However, this study did not differentiate the treatment effects of the vestibular compared with cervicogenic interventions that were combined into one treatment group. Therefore, it is impossible to determine whether the effects reported were attributable to one or both of these interventions. Regardless, this research provides tentative empirical support for the use of vestibular therapies in general. However, just as targeted treatments for concussion should match specific clinical profiles, so too should vestibular therapies match specific vestibular impairments and symptoms. Therefore, we review specific subtypes of vestibulospinal and vestibulo-ocular therapies in the sections that follow.

Vestibulospinal

Vestibulospinal dysfunction affects balance and gait performance. Although balance deficits following concussion often resolve spontaneously in the first few days following injury (Valovich McLeod & Hale, 2015), lingering postural instability affects some patients and may require therapy. Common therapies include sensory organization training involving alternating performance of balance with eyes closed, in different positions/ stances, on different surfaces, and while moving the head. Other effective approaches may involve dual tasks that require shifting attentional focus. For example, counting backwards numerically by sevens using three-digit numbers (i.e., serial 7s task) while balancing on a compliant foam pad will result in competing attentional demands. With regard to gait, a variety of physical therapies that target dynamic gait performance are used to restore gait function once postural stability is improved. Dual task gait performances such as walking while moving the head and tossing and catching a ball backwards may also be used to improve dynamic gait.

Vestibulo-Ocular

Vestibulo-ocular impairments, including vestibulo-ocular reflex impairment and sensitivity to visual movement or visually busy environments, are amenable to targeted vestibulo-ocular therapies. Among the more common exercises that the physical therapists in our clinic use to improve vestibulo-ocular reflex are those that improve gaze stability, or the eyes' ability to remain fixed on a visual target at the same time the head and/or body is moving. One example of this type of therapy is an exercise in which patients focus on a letter on an eye chart or piece of paper taped to the wall while simultaneously moving their head from side to side or up and down. An extension of this exercise might involve the patient performing the same task while walking toward or backing away from the chart. More advanced exercises may involve a patient focusing on a moving ball or object while shuffling back and forth in a "z" pattern on the floor. Exercises that target visual motion sensitivities (or space and motion discomfort) focus instead on graded exposure to increasing visually stimulating or challenging environments. For example, a patient may progress from walking down a hallway with its scrolling walls to walking through an open physical therapy clinic with its many simultaneous visual inputs. It is likely that these increasing exposures to busier visual environments may provoke symptoms. Consequently, patients should be closely monitored to adjust the exposure accordingly based on symptom provocation.

Many symptoms attributable to the vestibular system may actually have other underlying causes. As such, differential diagnoses are useful to help provide alternate explanations and guide subsequent targeted therapies. Dizziness in particular may arise from cervicogenic (i.e., neck related), preexisting migraine, and psychological factors. As a result, when vestibular therapies are ineffective in reducing symptoms such as dizziness and related impairments, other therapies that target the identified cause are needed. Cervicogenic causes of dizziness in particular are amenable to manipulative, proprioceptive, and ancillary therapies (Treleaven, 2011).

As with any specific treatment for concussion, only licensed health care professionals such as physical therapists trained in vestibular rehabilitation should prescribe and perform vestibular therapies.

Vision and Oculomotor Therapies

Vision therapies are becoming a more common component in the treatment toolkit for patients with concussion. However, there is very limited support in the literature for these therapies, with most of that support coming from a couple of studies with fairly small samples. Patients with oculomotor clinical profiles benefit from specialized vision training. A variety of oculomotor-related issues, such as convergence and accommodative insufficiencies, misalignments, and versional problems, can be mitigated with appropriate targeted vision therapies. As with vestibular therapies, vision therapies should be supervised by a licensed optometry or ophthalmology professional trained in concussion or neurobehavioral optometry.

One example of a simple oculomotor exercise that is often used to improve convergence-related impairment and symptoms is pencil push-ups, which involve focusing the eyes on a pencil held by a patient's arm at varying distances. Another exercise that is often used is the ladder beads (i.e., Brock strings), which involve focusing on beads on a string at different distances. Some more advanced exercises that target oculomotor impairment and symptoms use shifting of focus from near (e.g., a newspaper held in one's hand) to far (e.g., letters on an eye chart) objects (see Figure 5.1). One challenging way to facilitate this exercise is to have patients scan for progressive letters in the alphabet alternating between near and far locations. These types of exercises have positive transfer to reading and shifting attention in a classroom or work environment from near to far focus, for example, when a student in a math class is alternating focus between a textbook and the smart board or projector screen.

As alluded to above, the evidence for oculomotor and vision therapies in patients with concussion is very limited. Among the few published studies are several nonrandomized, retrospective trials that provide tentative support for the effectiveness of vision therapy on specific impairments following concussion. In a small retrospective study of patients following concussion, researchers indicated that a general vision therapy program that included versional, vergence and accommodative therapies resulted in improvements in symptoms and self-report reading performance (Thiagarajan, Ciuffreda, Capo-Aponte, Ludlam, & Kapoor, 2014). In another study, these benefits were reported to persist approximately 2 to 3 months following the intervention (Thiagarajan & Ciuffreda, 2015). Similarly, in another study of 12 patients following concussion, researchers reported that a targeted oculomotor rehabilitation program improved saccadic eye movements and vergence and accommodation (Thiagarajan & Ciuffreda, 2014). The patients in this study also reported improved overall reading following the intervention. As with other active interventions following concussion, researchers need to conduct larger, randomized trials of oculomotor and vision therapies that target the effects of each therapy on specific impairments.

THE EVOLVING ROLE OF PHARMACOLOGICAL INTERVENTIONS FOR CONCUSSION

The use of pharmacological interventions for treating concussion is not new. Numerous pharmacological interventions including cyclosporine, erythropoietin, levetiracetam (Browning et al., 2016), nicotinamide, and simvastatin, have shown promise in TBI animal models (Kochanek, Bramlett, Shear, et al., 2016). In fact, our colleagues at the University of Pittsburgh (Patrick Kochanek and C. Edward Dixon at the Safar Center for Resuscitation Research Traumatic Brain Injury Program) recently published the results of their systematic and well-controlled animal model research on pharmacological interventions for TBI in a special issue in the *Journal of Neurotrauma* (Volume 33, Issue 6). Although their results are focused on TBI, their methods provide an excellent blueprint for evaluating the effectiveness of pharmacological interventions in concussion. Despite the success

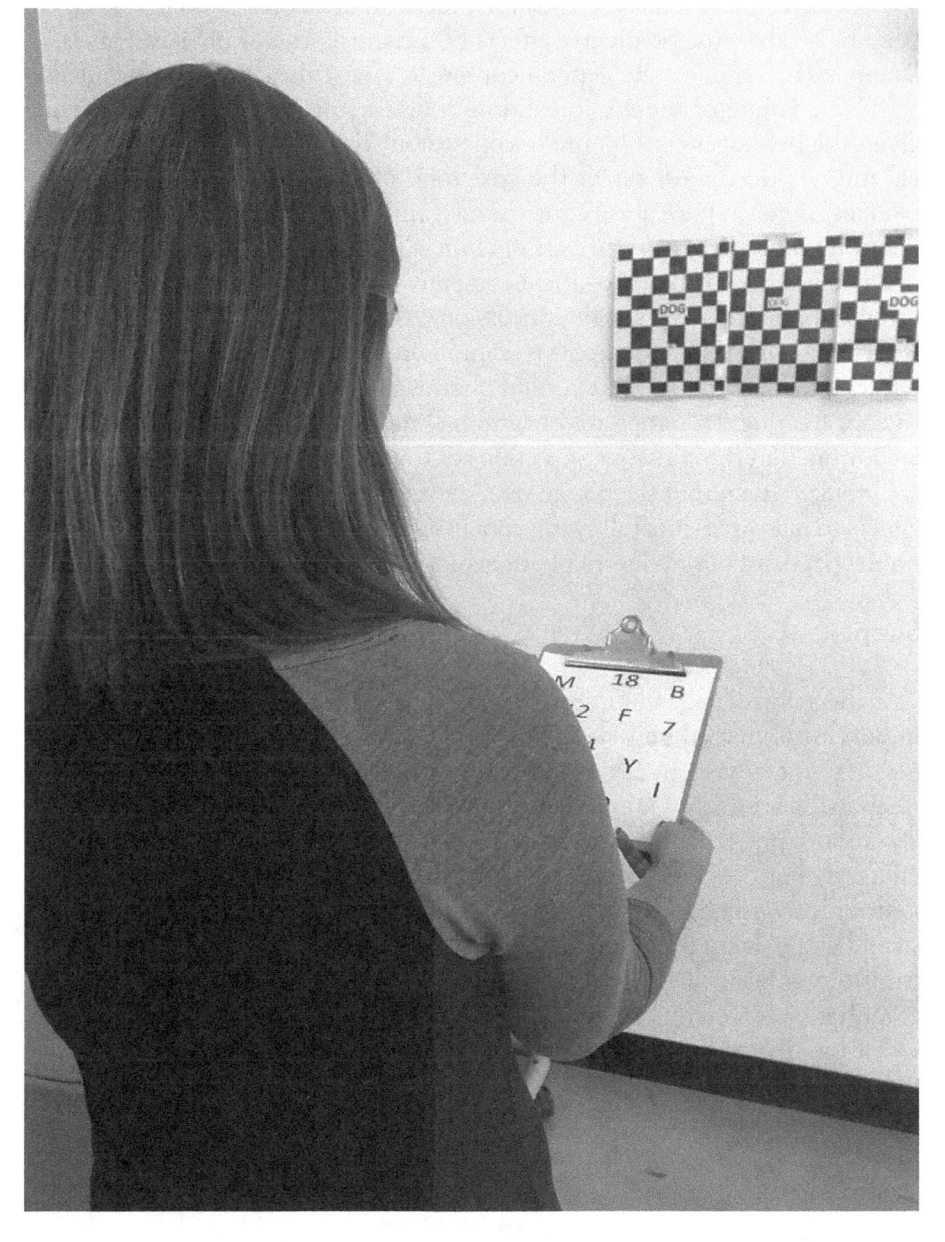

Figure 5.1. Shifting focus from near to far objects used to treat oculomotor impairment.

of some pharmacological interventions in animal models, most of the more than 200 clinical drug trials have focused on patients with moderate to severe TBI; none of these trials has met with measurable success, and several have been halted because of adverse effects (Z. Zhang, Larner, Kobeissy, Hayes, & Wang, 2010). In fact, the general consensus is that these trials have failed.

The failure of these clinical drug trials for concussion is not surprising given the heterogeneous nature of concussion. To be effective, pharmacological interventions must target the symptoms of specific clinical profiles. Any blanket approach to treating concussion using a general pharmacological intervention for all patients regardless of clinical profile is doomed to fail. Be wary of any clinician or pharmaceutical company touting a single pharmacological intervention for patients with concussion. Although empirical evidence from RCTs involving human patients is scant, there is mounting anecdotal and limited empirical evidence that certain pharmacological interventions are effective for treating the symptoms of certain clinical profiles. These interventions are outlined in the subsequent sections of this chapter and organized by clinical profile. Given that sleep is an overlay across all clinical profiles and that it affects so many patients following concussion, we also include a separate focus on sleep to start our review of pharmacological interventions for concussion.

Sleep

Because sleep is ubiquitous across patients with concussion, it is often important to first address sleep problems before targeting other clinical profiles. In our experience, many patients respond well to over-the-counter sleep medications, such as melatonin. Other pharmacological interventions commonly prescribed for sleep including zolpidem and eszopiclone can be effective, but they carry higher risks for dependency. Regardless of the intervention prescribed, we always include a sleep hygiene program to normalize sleep behaviors and maximize the effectiveness of prescribed pharmacological interventions. Researchers have advocated for this combined approach to enhance effects on sleep following concussion (e.g., Meehan, 2011). Occasionally, when other over-the-counter and prescription pharmacological interventions prove ineffective, some antidepressants, including amitriptyline, may be used to treat sleep problems.

Posttraumatic Migraine

The posttraumatic migraine (PTM) clinical profile is predictive of poor outcomes and longer recovery following concussion (Kontos, Elbin, Lau, et al., 2013). PTM symptoms (which typically include headache, nausea, and phono- or photo-sensitivity and may also include dizziness, vertigo, and vision-related symptoms) can be treated with a variety of pharmacological interventions. Among the more common pharmacological interventions used for PTM following concussion are antidepressants, including tricyclics (e.g., amitriptyline) and selective serotonin reuptake inhibitors (e.g., sertraline). In addition, anticonvulsants such as valproic acid and topiramate may be used. Triptans, which are referred to as *migraine abortive medications*, may also be used to treat PTM, but they should be used judiciously because of their potency and possible side effects, which may exacerbate other concussion-related symptoms, including fatigue, nausea, dizziness, and other types of headaches.

Cognitive Fatigue

Pharmacological interventions that stimulate the nervous system (i.e., neurostimulants) may be effective for treating the symptoms of cognitive fatigue, including memory problems, difficulty concentrating or paying attention, and increased fatigue and headaches as the day progresses. Among the more common neurostimulants is amantadine, which was developed as an antiviral to boost the immune response. We published a retrospective, historical controlled trial in adolescent patients that showed that amantadine was effective in reducing cognitive symptoms and impairments in memory and reaction time (Reddy, Collins, Lovell, & Kontos, 2013). Unfortunately, because of its generic nature, an RCT of amantadine for treating concussion has yet to be conducted. Despite this lack of evidence, amantadine is among the more commonly prescribed pharmacological interventions following concussion, with one in 10 clinicians reporting prescribing it (Kinnaman, Mannix, Comstock, & Meehan, 2013).

When amantadine is ineffective, patients may respond well to other neurostimulants, such as methylphenidate or Adderall. However, these more powerful neurostimulants tend to have increased side effects, including dizziness, anxiety, and sleep problems. (Note that amantadine may also exacerbate anxiety and cause or increase sleep problems but with less frequency and intensity than other neurostimulants.) In addition, some patients, particularly children, may already be on some medications such as Adderall for attention-deficit/hyperactivity disorder or other attentional problems. The use and effects of neurostimulants should be monitored closely, and dosage should be titrated appropriately to each patient and discontinued once the desired state has been attained.

Anxiety/Mood

The etiology of anxiety/mood in patients following concussion may relate to preexisting anxiety/mood issues, it may be a consequence of the psychosocial response to their concussion and its effects, or it may be a direct consequence from the injury to the brain itself. Regardless of the etiology, the treatment of patients who present with an anxiety/mood clinical profile following concussion is parallel in many respects to the treatment of patients with anxiety/mood issues without concussion. Both selective serotonin reuptake inhibitors (e.g., sertraline, paroxetine) and selective norepinephrine reuptake inhibitors (e.g., duloxetine) may be used with patients with anxiety/mood clinical profiles following concussion. Among the most commonly used pharmacological interventions for these patients is the tricyclic antidepressant amitriptyline, which may also be used to treat PTM and sleep problems following concussion.

All pharmacological interventions should be viewed as aggressive treatments that should be employed when the more conservative approaches described later in this chapter are ineffective. We believe strongly that with appropriate and timely behavioral interventions, and active therapies including exertion-based, vestibular, oculomotor, and vision, the need for pharmacological interventions can be mitigated. However, some patients may require a combination of active and pharmacological therapies for the best clinical outcome. We emphasize the importance of the multidisciplinary team approach to treating concussion when using pharmacological interventions.

Depending on which state one lives in, pharmacological interventions must be prescribed and supervised by clinicians who are licensed in that particular state. Regardless of who the prescriber is, information about dosage, possible treatment and side effects, and other relevant information should be shared among team members to provide for the most effective approach. Although patient responses to pharmacological interventions can be similar, individual patient variations can be significant and should be noted and generalized to inform subsequent pharmacological interventions for use with each clinical profile.

The review above is purposefully brief, intended to be an introduction to pharmacological interventions. The reader is encouraged to refer to more in-depth reviews of pharmacological interventions; see Brody (2014); Meehan (2011); and Petraglia, Maroon, and Bailes (2012).

TREATING PSYCHOLOGICAL ISSUES AFTER CONCUSSION

One of the biggest challenges for clinicians treating patients with concussion is psychological issues. They may be a direct result of the concussion or an indirect result of a psychological response to the injury and its concomitant isolation and unclear recovery trajectory (Kontos, Covassin, Elbin, & Parker, 2012). Psychological issues may also complicate recovery from concussion if not properly treated. At our clinic, we see patients at a variety of post-injury time points, from acute to chronic. Among patients who are referred or self-refer at a later (i.e., chronic) time from injury (e.g., a month or two following a concussion), many of them present with psychological sequelae, including anxiety and depressed mood. For these patients, the challenge is to disentangle the concussion-related symptoms from preexisting or secondary mood/anxiety symptoms. This process is challenging because of overlap in symptoms of anxiety, depression, and concussion (see Figure 3.1). To facilitate this, a detailed and thorough assessment of both pre- and postconcussion psychological wellness is needed (see Chapter 4). Ideally, as we have suggested (Covassin, Elbin, Larson, & Kontos, 2012), clinicians would have access to baseline assessments of psychological issues such as overall mood, depression, and anxiety. However, in their absence, a comprehensive psychological history using multiple sources (e.g., patient, parents, significant others) offers a reasonable proxy. Therefore, and similar to treatment for concussion clinical profiles, treatment for patients with psychological issues following concussion should be based on a comprehensive psychological assessment (see Chapter 4).

Treatment of psychological issues following concussion has received little attention in the literature. In fact, we recently completed one of the few published papers on the subject (Kontos, Deitrick, & Reynolds, 2016). Most of what has been published has focused on treating patients with post-concussion symptoms (e.g., Conder & Conder, 2015). Therefore, we begin by examining potential psychoeducational strategies to limit the psychological effects of concussion before it occurs. This primary prevention approach is designed to create a healthy level of baseline awareness of this injury, while also dispelling myths that often lead to fear in the absence of accurate and balance information on concussion.

Education/Awareness: Preventing Poor Outcomes and Setting Realistic Expectations

Although there is no way to completely prevent concussions from occurring, much can be done to educate patients prior to their injury that can help mitigate the effects of this injury. This information can also be extended to those involved with or affected by a patient with a concussion, including parents, coaches, military commanders, bosses, coworkers, and clinicians. Most important, patients, especially those at increased risk for concussion, such as young athletes in contact sports and certain military personnel, should be aware of the signs and symptoms of a concussion. In so doing, they might avoid long-term effects of this injury associated with delayed assessment and treatment. Moreover, awareness can help patients avoid potential, though rare, catastrophic effects of concussion from a second injury to the brain during the vulnerable period, such as second impact syndrome, as discussed in Chapter 2.

Most of the systematic efforts to improve awareness of concussion have been conducted in the context of sport, primarily within youth sport. In Pittsburgh, we initiated the Heads Up Pittsburgh concussion outreach program, which is designed to provide low cost or free neurocognitive baseline testing (using the ImPACT computerized testing system described in Chapter 4) as well as awareness and education about concussion to youth sport athletes and their parents. The program is conducted in locations that are convenient to athletes and their parents throughout the metropolitan Pittsburgh area. Athletes watch a 20-minute video on concussion awareness and then complete their baseline test, while their parents or guardians attend a live, 1-hour concussion educational seminar. This program is underwritten by the Pittsburgh Penguins Foundation, which is the philanthropic arm of the National Hockey League's Pittsburgh Penguins professional ice hockey team. To date, the Heads Up Pittsburgh program has provided testing and education/outreach on concussion to more than 12,000 youth sport athletes.

Empirical evidence for concussion awareness, education, and information is growing. In a systematic review of psychological approaches to treating concussion, researchers reported that providing information, reassurance, and education was more effective than no intervention in improving sleep, anxiety, and stress in three of nine published RCTs (Al Sayegh, Sandford, & Carson, 2010). However, six of the studies reported no effect for these interventions, and the focus of the research was on patients with postconcussion symptoms. A significant challenge for these awareness-based programs is to change not only knowledge but also attitudes and behaviors. In short, education and awareness programs are effective only insofar as they effect behavior change. After all, being aware of the signs and symptoms of concussion (i.e., knowledge) is a good start, but the ultimate objective of these efforts is to trigger a decision to remove oneself from military combat or a contact sport (i.e., behavior) because one might have a concussion. Moving forward, programs should assess how effective they are in changing behaviors like reporting concussion or seeking care in order to have the greatest impact on secondary prevention of concussion.

The second way in which psychoeducational strategies can be used is in the early postconcussion phase when patients are uncertain. These strategies may be particularly helpful to patients who have no direct or indirect experience with concussion. However, do not assume that these previous experiences necessarily have a positive effect on a patient's subsequent experiences with concussion. In fact, depending on the nature and outcomes of the previous experience, the opposite may be true. We have noticed that patients who have had previous negative experiences such as misdiagnosis, ineffective treatment, or setbacks during recovery often have a negative expectation following a subsequent concussion. This expectation may also hold true for a patient whose teammate or friend had a poor experience following a concussion. Therefore, clinicians need to qualify previous concussion experience—especially longer recoveries—with additional specifics about the nature of the experience itself. Note that an overemphasis on symptoms and the effects of concussion may have the paradoxical effect of increasing perceptions related to concussion, thereby making things worse for a patient. Therefore, clinicians need to balance their patients' need for information with the need to limit continued focus on their symptoms.

Cognitive Behavioral Therapies

In our experience, patients with anxiety/mood clinical profiles benefit from cognitive and behavioral management approaches. In our clinic, we use an approach that focuses on stress management, promotion of physical activity, and monitoring and regulation of sleep, nutrition, and hydration (see Figure 5.2). Concurrently, patients should avoid excessive alcohol and recreational and prescription drug use. Ancillary talk therapy and discussion of the nature of psychological issues following a concussion is also useful to help identify the source of the issues and better direct treatments. The evidence supporting the use of cognitive behavioral therapies (CBTs) in patients with concussion is small but consistent. In a systematic review of the literature of psychological treatments for postconcussion symptoms, Al Sayegh and colleagues (2010) reported that CBT approaches enhanced psychosocial functioning over routine care approaches. Effects attributed to CBT include a reduction in concussion symptoms, anxiety, and depression.

CBTs are often used in conjunction with other therapies, thereby making it difficult to determine the extent to which they are responsible for positive effects reported by patients. In addition, specific types of CBT strategies are not compared, so we do not know which of these strategies provide the greatest therapeutic benefit to patients. In-depth and long-term psychotherapy is an infrequently used approach for most patients following concussion; in our clinic, its use is largely restricted to patients with chronic symptoms and those with pervasive or worsening psychological issues that are not amenable to more commonly used CBT and other brief therapies.

IMPORTANCE OF COPING AND SOCIAL SUPPORT

The ways in which a patient deals with a concussion, including both the direct effects of the injury itself (e.g., symptoms, impairment) and the concomitant effects on their daily life (e.g., personal, social, work/academic),

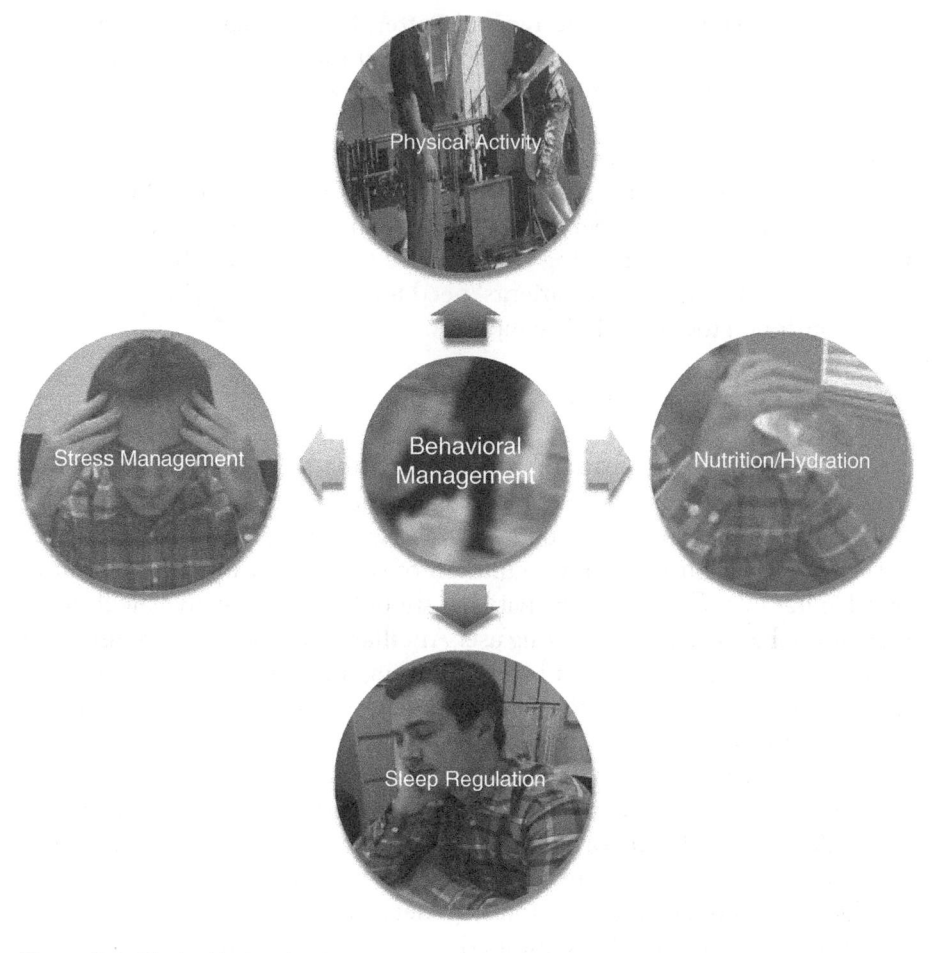

Figure 5.2. Typical behavioral management components for patients with a concussion.

can play a substantial role in mitigating or even preventing altogether the psychological issues associated with this injury. Coping may include both emotion-focused (i.e., regulating emotional distress) and problem-focused (i.e., engaging in actions to improve emotional distress) approaches (Folkman & Lazarus, 1985). Coping can also be viewed as adaptive or positive in nature or maladaptive or negative. For example, a patient may cope with the negative feelings of not being with her classmates following a concussion by avoiding all contact with them while injured (i.e., problem-focused, maladaptive). Another patient may cope with the same situation by seeking information about recovery from her teammates who previously had a concussion (i.e., problem-focused, adaptive).

A common form of coping is social support, involving both tangible and intangible support provided by others including family, friends, teammates/coworkers, teachers/bosses, and health care providers. Social support may take the form of listening, emotional, task-related, personal, or financial support (Richman, Rosenfeld, & Hardy, 1993). Researchers have reported that social support can increase adherence (Evans, Hardy, & Fleming, 2000) and reduce isolation and fear of reinjury following orthopedic injuries (Podlog & Eklund, 2004).

Given that both social support and coping play a positive role in dealing with injury and minimizing the negative psychological effects associated with injury (Clement & Shannon, 2011), it stands to reason that they would have the same positive effects on patients following concussion, especially for those already dealing with psychological issues following their injury. However, concussions are unlike orthopedic and other injuries in that the evidence of them is less overt, they have a more inconsistent (patient to patient) recovery trajectory, and they have historically involved inactive approaches to treatment. As such, social support and coping, while potentially equally important to help patients following a concussion as following any other injury, may not be used or experienced in the same way after a concussion. Moreover, athletes may not cope the same way as nonathletes. However, research on coping with concussion is limited to sport environments.

A handful of studies on coping following concussion have suggested that concussion may elicit different coping responses than other types of injuries. Woodrome and colleagues (2011) examined coping in children with concussion and those with orthopedic injuries and found that coping accounted for 10% to 15% of the variance in reported symptoms. These researchers also reported that emotion-focused coping was related to higher concussion symptoms and that problem-focused coping might moderate symptoms following a concussion. Similarly, we studied athletes with concussion or orthopedic injuries and uninjured controls and found that concussed athletes reported lower levels of coping than the other groups (Kontos, Elbin, Newcomer Appaneal, Covassin, & Collins, 2013). In fact, following a concussion, athletes coped very little, which may reflect uncertainty about coping with an invisible injury. In contrast, because a concussion often results in prescribed rest and inactivity, patients with a concussion may consciously decide not to cope immediately following injury. In this same study, we found that females were more likely than males to vent, plan, use humor, and seek instrumental support following concussion. This finding suggests that factors such as sex and age may play a role in coping and its effectiveness following a concussion.

Researchers have reported that following a concussion, athletes experience emotional disturbance and may benefit from social support (Mainwaring, Hutchison, Bisschop, Comper, & Richards, 2010). However, research on social support following concussion is limited to a single study. In that study, Covassin and colleagues (2014) reported that concussed athletes and athletes with orthopedic injuries reported similar sources of social support, including family, friends, teammates, and sports medicine professionals. This finding highlights the potentially impactful role of sports medicine and other health care professionals in providing social support to patients following a concussion. However, the researchers also found that the concussed athletes did not report the same level of satisfaction with support from these sources. Even though both groups relied on the same sources for support, the concussed group may not have benefitted the same as the group with orthopedic injuries. This finding may be related to the fact that people do not know how to respond to someone with a concussion, which, unlike an orthopedic injury, is invisible and lacks overt evidence of injury beyond symptoms and impairment (Bloom et al., 2004). Therefore, it is important to leverage support from the most salient sources of social support, including family and significant others.

Leveraging Family and Significant Others

Given the importance of social support outlined in the preceding section and the fact that family and significant others represent a substantial source of social support, their potential positive contribution to the recovery process following concussion is considerable. However, not all support provided by family and significant others results in positive outcomes for patients with a concussion. Our offices are right outside of the waiting room, and we can often gauge parents' and others' level of support prior to seeing the patient. The level of support runs the spectrum from being completely supportive (perhaps even too much so; see the next section) to being completely disengaged or unsupportive to the point of telling the patient the problem is "all in their head." (It is unclear whether they intend the pun.) Lack of support can erode the foundation set by the health care professionals during the initial and subsequent appointments because patients have limited contact with the health care professional but constant contact with family or significant others. Therefore, it is important to enlist, and cultivate if necessary, the support of these individuals.

One strategy that can be effective in gaining buy-in from family and significant others is to provide them with suggestions for overt roles or tasks (i.e., tangible support) to assist in the recovery process. For example, a family member can pick up missed assignments and communicate with teachers or employers. Even younger family members can help by encouraging the patient to complete their rehabilitation exercises or by going on a walk with the patient in the early phases of exertion therapy. Another strategy that has shown to be effective is to have family members provide emotional support through positive and occasional brief discussions of the injury process. These discussions should focus on what the patient can control and positive steps that they can take moving forward. It is important to note that family support should be consistent, occasional, and balanced in order to avoid potential negative effects from overinvolved family members that constantly inquire about symptoms or repeatedly ask, "How are you feeling?" As we discuss in the next section, good intentions do not always result in positive outcomes for the patient and in some cases may actually make things worse.

A Caveat About Helicopter Parents

There is a well-worn saying in our clinic: "You can tell if a kid is going to do poorly with this injury based on the thickness of the binder their parents bring in with them to the appointment." With the easy availability of information from the Internet, these parents often arrive armed with multiple sources of concussion information and have already diagnosed their child. Yes, these aptly named "helicopter parents"—who exert significant control over their children and often direct their responses during the clinical interview—can play a significant role in the assessment, treatment, and recovery processes for young patients with a concussion. In fact, research suggests that hyperparenting can even adversely affect a child's physical activity (Janssen, 2015). Although there is no empirical evidence yet, we have observed strong anecdotal evidence that this parenting style may affect concussion outcomes. In particular, it seems to increase anxiety/mood responses and promote a hypervigilance for symptoms among patients. One might assume that helicopter parenting would only affect children; however, the effects appear to extend well into a child's entry into adulthood (Fingerman et al., 2012). We have seen many college-aged and young adults who have been accompanied to their concussion appointments with a parent. Although these helicopter parents may appear to be a hindrance to recovery, they can also be recruited to help promote compliance with rehabilitation programs.

Sleep Interventions

After a concussion, sleep is important to both the brain recovery process and the general psychological well-being of the patient. Sleep interventions may be warranted when a patient experiences psychological sequelae following injury. Sleep interventions may occur in the acute phase immediately following injury or further down the line. Early postinjury interventions should target awareness and development of good sleep habits to minimize the risk of subsequent sleep disorders (Wickwire et al., 2016). These early interventions are built on sound education regarding sleep quality for the patient and those around them. This education should focus first on awareness and then on the development of good sleep habits. Monitoring of sleep using journals or smartphone and sleep tracker technology may be useful for some patients to provide awareness of their disturbed sleep. However, an overemphasis on monitoring sleep may have the paradoxical effect of worsening sleep as a result of the hyperawareness, so moderation is the key.

Patients should also learn how to apply specific strategies for improving sleep quality, including consistent timing of sleep; avoidance of technology at sleep time; and the effects of food, caffeine, and alcohol on sleep. The goal of these interventions is to minimize the effects of concussion on the sleep–wake cycle, which can have a detrimental effect on recovery, as well as psychological issues. Further out from injury, patients may adopt more pervasive (though less effective) sleep patterns of hypersomnia. This pattern of sleeping more than usual can exacerbate symptoms such as fatigue and lack of energy and serve as an ineffective avoidance coping strategy. Health care professionals should instead encourage regular sleep schedules of normalized (6–9 hours) duration. Taking multiple naps throughout the day should also be discouraged. For more information about sleep interventions and the effects of concussion on sleep, see Wickwire et al. (2016).

EMERGING APPROACHES TO TREATING PSYCHOLOGICAL ISSUES RELATED TO CONCUSSION

The psychological treatment approaches described previously represent what can loosely be referred to as more established therapies for treating psychological issues related to concussion. However, several emerging therapies have recently begun to gain momentum. Although only limited or even no evidence supports these therapies at the current time, they warrant discussion because they might augment current approaches and they have intuitive appeal to patients with this injury.

Mindfulness

In the only empirical study to date on mindfulness with concussion, Azulay and colleagues (2013) examined the effects of a mindfulness program in 22 individuals with chronic (i.e., > 7 months) postconcussion symptoms. The intervention consisted of a modified version of the mindfulness-based stress reduction program developed by Kabat-Zinn and colleagues (1998; Kabat-Zinn et al., 1992) in a number of studies, with additional attention-based and awareness of internal and external experience related to acceptance and attitude. They found a strong effect for both improved quality of life and perceived self-efficacy following the mindfulness intervention. Smaller effects suggested that both attention and working memory also improved. However, this study did not include a control group, so any effects reported may have occurred spontaneously. In an early RCT of mindfulness in patients with a range of TBI from mild to moderate, researchers concluded that mindfulness had no effect (McMillan et al., 2002). Most mindfulness approaches combine being mindful with relaxation strategies, making it difficult to ascertain which strategy is responsible for the reported effects. Some clinicians believe that mindfulness may be harmful to some patients through an over-awareness of symptoms, particularly for those who are already fixated on their symptoms. Therefore, although mindfulness may be useful in some patients, it may not be effective for certain patients (e.g., somaticizers).

Art, Music, and Pet Therapies

At the National Intrepid Center of Excellence brain injury treatment center in Bethesda, Maryland, active duty military personnel with a protracted concussion or TBI complete an intensive 4-week comprehensive and immersive treatment program. The program includes extensive neuroimaging and clinical assessments and interviews together with multidisciplinary approaches to treatment involving cognitive rehabilitation, vestibular and physical therapies, vision therapies, and pharmacological treatments. In addition, the program augments these more traditional approaches to treating concussion with art, music, and pet therapies. The art therapy, which was featured on a recent episode of the television news program 60 Minutes, focuses on expressing the emotional side of their concussion and other comorbid issues (e.g., posttraumatic stress, substance abuse) through sculpture. The focus of this therapy is on the creation of a facial mask that represents the patient's feelings related to their injury. We have seen the masks; they are powerful to look at and must have a cathartic effect for patients. Music therapy is also used. Patients are encouraged to play instruments and use music as a form of expressing their feelings associated with their injury. Some patients even formed a band as part of their music therapy; regular practices and jam sessions give patients a release and might facilitate the recovery process.

One of the more interesting aspects of the treatment program at the Bethesda facility is the opportunity for patients to have contact with specially trained service animals. Becoming overly reliant on a pet for support can have potential adverse effects, including lack of ownership for one's recovery, but these interactions are particularly useful for military personnel who may have a hard time opening up about their injury to clinicians. During a visit to the facility, we had the opportunity to see a patient interact with a companion dog who served as a nonjudgmental listener. During this interaction the patient's eyes lit up and his demeanor went from quiet and guarded to laughter and openness. He even began talking to the dog about his injury and where he was in the recovery process. Although programs that use art, music, and pet therapies are not the norm for treating the psychological issues associated with concussion, these therapies along with mindfulness approaches are likely to become more common in the future. As they do, we need a concomitant increase in empirical research to determine their effectiveness.

A Brief Note About Referrals

When psychological issues are identified and especially when they become more pronounced, clinicians should consider a referral for specialized mental health care. In a clinic such as ours, which uses a sports medicine model predicted on rapid team-based intervention, it is easy to facilitate referrals to specialists in any number of areas, as described in Chapter 1. Ideally, a clinician working alone in private practice will also have cultivated a referral network to cover different psychological issues, such as anxiety, depression, adjustment disorder, and conversion disorder, that are beyond their scope of expertise. We have had many referrals of patients who were managed by a single provider who attempted to wear too many hats and ended up providing subpar or no care at all for psychological issues related to a patient's concussion. Obviously, this is an extreme example, but it highlights the importance of knowing when to refer and having the appropriate referral network in place.

DETERMINING SAFE RETURN TO ACTIVITY: A MODIFIED APPROACH

Ultimately, concussion recovery is determined on the basis of a patient's ability to return to full or normal activities. Any patient who is unable to return to full activity following a concussion is considered to have lingering symptoms or impairment (referred to as *postconcussion symptoms* or *postconcussion syndrome*; P. McCrory et al., 2013). Current published clinical guidelines for return to activity—which is referred to as *return to play* in sport and *return to duty* in the military—recommend that patients be asymptomatic and back to baseline level of cognitive, balance, or other assessed impairments at rest and that they be asymptomatic following exertion (P. McCrory et al., 2013). The current consensus on return to activity has been based primarily on return to play guidelines from sport-related consensus guidelines. As such, these guidelines may require additional customization for use with military and nonathlete populations. Although the intent of return to activity guidelines is to promote safe return to activity that prevents the exacerbation of the current injury, the current guidelines are flawed in several respects. Most important, the guidelines rely heavily on symptom reporting, which does not reflect impairment (cognitive, vestibular, oculomotor, balance) per se.

With regard to being asymptomatic, not all patients bring the same baseline level of symptoms to the table. In a recent study, we found that 11% of patients report high levels of baseline symptoms, and on average, patients report symptom severity scores on the Post-Concussion Symptom Scale (Lovell & Collins, 1998) of about 6, but with a larger variability ($SD = 12$; Custer et al., 2016). Although a clinician may not have access to baseline symptom scores, other factors can be used to identify patients who might report higher levels of symptoms in general that would not necessarily be related to their concussion. In a study involving 120 pediatric patients seen at the emergency department, patients with high somatization scores were more likely to take longer to recover based on symptoms, and females were more likely to be somaticizers and report prolonged symptoms following a concussion (Root et al., 2016). Although this finding may intimate that these patients experience worse effects following a concussion, it is likely that they simply have higher baseline levels of symptoms related to concussion (regardless of injury status) and other maladies for that matter.

Because current guidelines are limited to specific populations, we recommend that clinicians augment the current approach with several key components: (a) postexertion assessments of cognitive, balance, or other assessed impairments; (b) dynamic exertion protocol; and (c) clinical profile–based return to activity determination. In so doing, clinicians will help to ensure that their patients are ready to return to the specific activities of their daily lives in the safest manner possible. Each of the components is described in the sections that follow.

Postexertion Assessments of Impairment

We believe that it is important to assess symptoms following exertion protocols, but this approach alone falls short. As discussed above and supported in the study by McGrath and colleagues (2013), patients' reported symptoms do not always match up with postexertion levels of impairment. In short, if we rely solely on self-reported symptoms following exertion, we are likely to return to activity many (up to 33.3% per the McGrath et al. findings) patients who are not yet ready to do so. Therefore, we suggest the implementation of postexertion cognitive, balance, and other testing to identify patients who might not report symptoms but do experience exacerbated impairment following exertion. Research suggests that testing immediately following exertion can influence performance on cognitive (Covassin, Weiss,

Powell, Womack, & Lovell, 2007) and balance (Fox, Mihalik, Blackburn, Battaglini, & Guskiewicz, 2008) tests in healthy individuals, and so we recommend that any such testing occur after a 5- to 10-minute rest period.

Although there is no research on the topic, it is possible that the assessment of symptoms immediately following exertion may result in elevated symptoms related to the exertion rather than the concussion per se. However, more research in this area is needed before we change the current approach. Additionally, many symptoms that are reported following aerobic exertion may relate more to baseline levels of aerobic fitness or reductions in aerobic fitness levels from physical inactivity following a concussion, than from the concussion itself. Furthermore, the use of aerobic exertion involving cycling and treadmill running may not sufficiently exert patients with certain clinical profiles, such as vestibular, to elicit symptoms. As such, additional exertion protocols may be warranted to flesh out symptoms for patients with certain clinical profiles.

Dynamic Exertion Protocol

One additional approach to assessing return to activity involves the use of dynamic exertion protocols. In our clinic, we have developed what we affectionately call the Exertional Test (EXiT) protocol. The protocol was developed by our physical therapist, Cara Troutman-Enseki, DPT, in conjunction with our clinical faculty. The EXiT consists of both a cardiovascular assessment and a dynamic exertion circuit. It begins with the cardiovascular component, and if patients are able to tolerate 30 minutes of moderate intensity activity (e.g., running, cycling, elliptical) in accordance with American College of Sports Medicine guidelines, then they progress to the dynamic exertion component. The dynamic exertion component includes multiple repetitions of whole body movements such as medicine ball rotations and lunges. If patients are able to complete this component without symptoms or impairment, then they move to the function component of the EXiT. The functional component is activity specific and is designed to simultaneously tax the cardiovascular, vestibular, and visual systems. Licensed physical therapists conduct the ExiT and periodically (i.e., before and after each component) monitor heart rate, blood pressure, concussion symptom provocation, and vestibular and oculomotor symptom provocation and impairment throughout the protocol (see Figure 5.3).

The goal of this dynamic exertion-based evaluation is to ensure that our patients are truly ready to return to the activities to which they aspire. Therefore, we conduct an exertion protocol that includes a combination of both aerobic and dynamic exertion. Our approach is somewhat in contrast to the one advocated by expert consensus, which involves a return to full

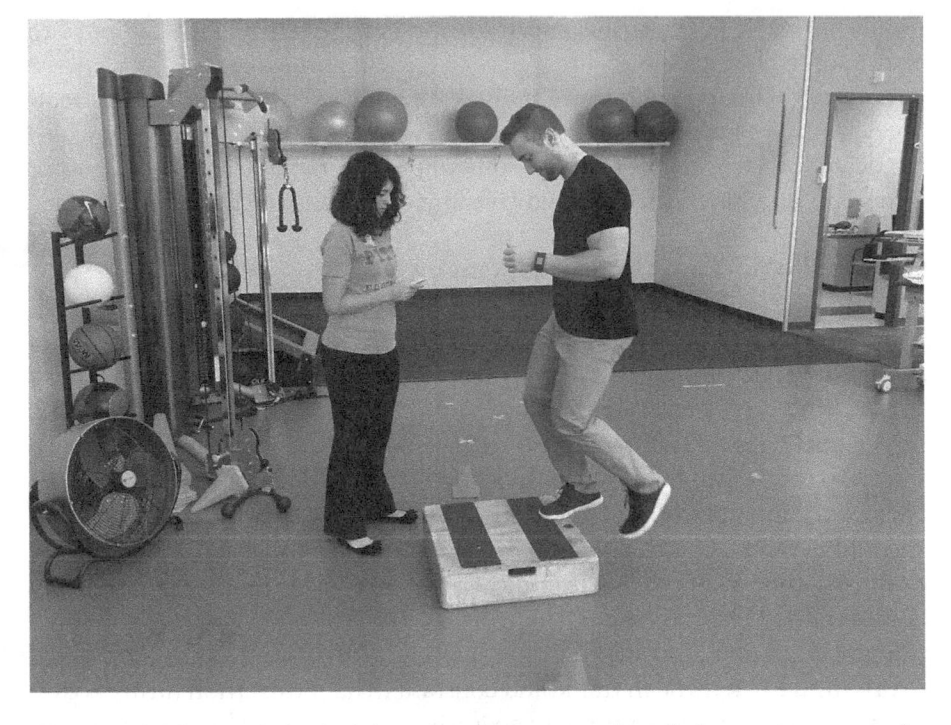

Figure 5.3. A licensed physical therapist monitors a patient during a component of the dynamic exertion component of the Exertional Test.

activity through a series of five to six progressive stages of exposure to increases in exertion—from no activity to full return to activity—based largely on cardiovascular demands (e.g., McCrory et al., 2013, 2017). Although the stepwise progression promoted in the Concussion in Sport Group consensus documents promotes some sport-specific dynamic movements, there is no systematic approach, and the focus is primarily on aerobic exertion.

In practice, this approach typically requires 5 to 7 days of progression, as long as a patient does not report increased symptoms following any particular stage or step along the way. Leddy and Willer (2013) suggested that such a graded approach, if based on heart rate and reported symptoms, can be effective in determining readiness for return to activity. In their research, Leddy and Willer relied on a treadmill and running (i.e., the Buffalo Concussion Treadmill Test) to determine readiness to return to normal activity. However, this approach assumes a linear progression and also that all patients will respond the same way to increases in cardiovascular demand. In our experience, this assumption is not always accurate; any number of factors, from baseline cardiovascular fitness to concussion clinical profile, may influence performance. Instead, the progression should take into account the clinical profiles of each patient, the nature of the activity to which they plan to return, and when possible, differences in baseline fitness levels. As such, we advocate for an approach that involves dynamic exertion that mimics real-life activities, especially for patients with vestibular clinical profiles. We also advocate for assessment of concussion symptoms, vestibular and oculomotor symptoms and function, and cognitive function following these movements.

Clinical Profile–Based Return to Activity

The driving force behind any determination of return to full activity should be based on the individual patient's specific situation. For example, a patient who drives a delivery truck in heavy city traffic and loads and unloads heavy packages all day long on a tight time schedule needs to be able to return to those specific activities in a safe manner; similarly, a patient who is an accountant and works at a desk all day on numerical calculation involving spreadsheets on a computer must be able to return to those activities. In both examples, the patient's specific clinical profile will drive the return to activity determination. In the case of the delivery driver, a concussion involving a primary vestibular clinical profile may present a different challenge for return to driving a truck through traffic and constant dynamic exertion lifting boxes; a concussion involving a primary cognitive-fatigue clinical profile may present less of a challenge to returning to these activities. In summary, clinicians should always consider the clinical profiles in the context of the patient's daily preconcussion activities when determining a safe return to activity. Although safe determination of return to full activity is important for all patients, it is particularly important for patients who are returning to sport or military duty because these activities carry a high risk of recurrent injury and potential, though rare, catastrophic injury.

FOLLOW-UP CARE: MONITORING THE EFFECTS OF CONCUSSION AND ADJUSTING TREATMENT

Coordination of follow-up care is critical to the successful treatment of patients with concussion. Coordinating clinicians should also maintain close contact with the follow-up providers, who are often the same providers who referred patients for treatment. We believe that follow-up is particularly important to determine patient compliance with rehabilitation and prescribed medications and to help monitor medication side effects, patient improvement, and potential lingering symptoms and deficits. However, follow-up should not entail constant symptom evaluation and discussion of the injury; doing so may have the paradoxical effect of increasing symptoms as a result of hyperawareness and focus. A good rule of thumb is to monitor and follow up every 5 to 7 days early in the injury process and 7 to 10 days later on.

Follow-up care does not necessarily mean face-to-face care. Follow-up care may be provided by phone, via the web, and via smartphone. Recently we have been conducting research involving the use of PT Pal, which provides a patient interface to support our active physical therapy interventions through a smartphone application. These e-platforms for follow-up will continue to expand as the technology and support become more established.

We would expect follow-up care to benefit patients, but that may not always be the case. Somewhat surprisingly, researchers reported that a randomized trial of a phone counseling follow-up intervention at 1-week and 1-month intervals following discharge from the emergency department was ineffective in reducing symptoms in pediatric patients (Mortenson, Singhal, Hengel, & Purtzki, 2016). However, in this study the intervention, which focused on reviewing symptom and return to activity, may have inadvertently resulted in parents and their children overfocusing on their symptoms, which was the outcomes variable.

In contrast, in a preliminary study of 13 adolescents with concussion, researchers reported that a web-based intervention that focused on activity monitoring and relaxation may be effective in reducing symptoms and increasing activity following concussion (Kurowski et al., 2016). However, more research is needed; this study did not include a control group, and the sample was very small. Periodic follow-up of some kind is likely beneficial to patients following concussion, especially those with lingering symptoms and impairment.

CONCLUSION

Treatment for patients with concussion should flow from the clinical profiles identified during the comprehensive assessment and be targeted to the most problematic profile. Under ideal conditions, patients with concussion will be treated by an interdisciplinary team coordinated by a clinician.

Despite perceptions to the contrary, rest is not the only treatment for concussion, and more active approaches are gaining empirical support. In fact, rest may do more harm than good for some patients. Strict rest or cocoon therapy is never indicated for patients with concussion. Other active, targeted approaches to treatment, including exertion, vestibular, oculomotor, and vision therapies, may enhance recovery following concussion. In some cases, patients may benefit from pharmacological interventions that target specific clinical profiles. Psychological treatments may be needed for some patients, especially those further out from injury, and should flow from a comprehensive assessment and ideally, from information about preinjury psychological health. Educational strategies, CBT, sleep interventions, coping, and social support can all help patients dealing with psychological issues following a concussion. However, be aware of hypersupportive helicopter parents; they can have unintended negative effects on young patients.

Emerging treatments, including mindfulness, art, and music, may be effective for some patients with psychological issues following concussion. Additional research on the effectiveness of these and other treatment strategies for psychological issues related to concussion are needed. Occasionally, specialized referrals for psychotherapy and more targeted treatment for underlying psychological issues following concussion are indicated. Regardless of the type of treatment, additional research involving RCTs with humans is needed to understand which therapies work with which patients. Determining safe return to activity is important and should incorporate postexertion cognitive testing, comprehensive exertion protocols that include both cardiovascular and dynamic components, and be specific to patient clinical profiles and day-to-day activities. Follow-up care is the final piece in the treatment puzzle, without which successful treatment outcomes for patients will be challenging.

6

CASE STUDIES

In this chapter, we present three cases that highlight the clinical profiles, comprehensive assessment, and targeted treatments discussed in the preceding chapters. The purpose of this chapter is to illustrate how the initial presentation, injury information, medical and psychosocial history, and clinical findings are used to inform clinical profile(s) and targeted treatments (see Chapters 1 and 5, respectively) to enhance the recovery of each patient. In so doing, we also consider the injury information, including signs, symptoms, and impairment, together with relevant primary and secondary risk factors (see Chapter 2). We integrate into this information the outcomes from the comprehensive assessment approach (Chapter 4). Where applicable we also highlight psychological issues (from Chapter 3) and concomitant interventions (from Chapter 5) used in each case. The objective of this chapter is to apply all of the information from the preceding chapters to real-life cases similar to those that professionals and students may encounter in their practices, research, or training.

http://dx.doi.org/10.1037/0000087-007
Concussion: A Clinical Profile Approach to Assessment and Treatment, by A. P. Kontos and M. W. Collins
Copyright © 2018 by the American Psychological Association. All rights reserved.

FORMAT FOR CASE STUDIES

Each case is organized chronologically from initial clinical visit to final outcome. We describe patients who presented initially in the acute, subacute, and chronic phases of concussion. Each case study represents an actual patient whose demographic data have been changed to protect anonymity. However, the main clinical presentations, symptoms, impairment, clinical profiles, targeted treatments, and outcomes are consistent with the actual cases. Much as is the case in our clinic, each of these cases represents multiple clinical profiles. Although we acknowledge that some patients present with a single clinical profile, it is far more common for patients to present with multiple clinical profiles that require prioritization, as the cases presented here illustrate. Therefore, we indicate which profiles are primary, secondary, or tertiary where applicable for each patient. Profiles are depicted using circles that correspond in size to the primary, secondary, and tertiary classifications and include supporting findings as well as targeted treatments that were implemented with each patient.

We discuss relevant medical and psychosocial histories for each patient as well as any key injury information. Often, we see patients weeks or months after injury, and their symptoms and impairment may have changed over that time. As such, we also include descriptions of both signs and symptoms at the time of injury, as well as those that are current when the patient presents to the clinic. We then explore the findings from the clinical interview/exams, symptoms, computerized neurocognitive tests (CNTs), vestibular and oculomotor screening, and exertional testing, as well as any additional testing or referrals for further evaluation. Next, we describe the case conceptualization using the appropriate clinical profiles with supporting information. We then discuss prescribed treatments, referrals, and interventions, followed by the disposition of the case. For each case, we include a figure that visually depicts the connection between the risk factors, symptoms, and impairment; clinical profiles; and subsequent targeted treatments. Throughout the various phases of each case, we highlight the roles of specialist members of the clinical treatment team when applicable.

In our clinic and the cases described here, the clinical neuropsychologist serves as the "point guard" who conducts the initial assessment and referrals and coordinates care throughout the recovery process. Other clinics may have different health care professionals in this role or may rely on only one clinician because of geographical, financial, and other limitations. Regardless of who or how many individuals are involved in a patient's care, consultation and referrals with experts in specific domains (e.g., vestibular physical therapist, behavioral neuro-optometrist, physicians) offer the most effective and efficient path forward to recovery. We conclude each case with a summary of the outcomes and follow-up information.

CASE 1. CONSEQUENCES OF CONTINUING TO PLAY
WHILE SYMPTOMATIC

Initial Presentation

Nick is a 14-year-old American boy who presents to the clinic 5 days after sustaining a concussion during a football game. His primary complaints are dizziness with movement, imbalance, and persistent daily bitemporal headache with nausea. He was initially evaluated on-field at the end of his game by a certified athletic trainer (ATC) who reported that his initial symptoms included headache, dizziness, nausea, and bilateral blurred vision. After a few minutes on the sideline, Nick also began reporting photosensitivity and fatigue. He hid his symptoms and continued to play for about 20 to 30 minutes until the game ended. It was only after the game that he went to the ATC to be evaluated.

Injury Information

Nick reports a head-to-head collision with an opposing player away from the play during a block. Because the play occurred away from the action/ball, no one on the sideline or field recognized the injury. He reports feeling wobbly, dizzy, and off balance and having trouble seeing straight (immediate symptoms). Despite his awareness of his symptoms, he decides to hide them and continue to play, because, as in his words, "it was a playoff game." He reports no loss of consciousness, posttraumatic amnesia, disorientation, or confusion at the time of injury. He says he did not notice his symptoms again until the game was over, at which time he felt very dizzy, had trouble walking off the field straight, and had a headache on both sides of his head.

Medical and Psychosocial History

Nick reports a history of five previous concussions during the past 2 years. He also reports continuing to play following two of these concussions despite his awareness of symptoms. Academically, prior to his concussions he reports being an A (i.e., excellent) student, whereas currently his grades are Bs and Cs (i.e., average). He has no other personal medical or psychosocial history to report. However, his father indicates during the initial exam that he (the father) has had migraine headaches since he was about 17 to 18 years old.

Clinical Findings

In addition to the dizziness, imbalance, and headaches, Nick reports feeling foggy, intermittent blurry vision, dizziness while walking down the hallway at school, fatigue, and sleep problems. His total symptom severity score on the Post-Concussion Symptom Scale (PCSS; Lovell & Collins, 1998) is 34, reflecting a moderate symptom presentation. Dizziness and headache are his primary symptoms, but he also reports sleeping less and having memory problems. The only affective related symptom that he reports is irritability. His CNT results indicate significant impairment on visual memory (< 1st percentile) and reaction time (9th percentile), with moderate impairment on verbal memory (26th percentile) and visual motor processing speed (46th percentile). Nick's most pronounced impairment is evidenced in his symptom provocation following the vestibular components of the Vestibular/Ocular Motor Screening (VOMS) assessment. Specifically, his vestibulo-ocular reflex (VOR) and visual motion sensitivity (VMS) scores are 6 (out of 10) for dizziness and nausea. His near point convergence (NPC) distance is at 4 centimeters (i.e., normal), and his pursuits and saccades were unremarkable for symptoms. As a result of his substantial dizziness with movement and significant headache, we do not conduct exertional testing with Nick. A physical medicine and rehabilitation physician conducts a cervical evaluation, on which he tests negative.

Referrals and Additional Testing

As a result of the VOMS, Nick is referred to a vestibular physical therapist for follow-up vestibular assessment to determine which components of the vestibular system are impaired. He tests negative for benign paroxysmal positional vertigo (BPPV), which is caused by the otoconia being dislodged into the semicircular canals. The vestibular physical therapist performs both the Dix-Hallpike and supine roll tests, which are screening tests using head movements to rule out BPPV. In additional testing, Nick performs poorly on the dynamic visual acuity test and reports significant, provoked dizziness during and after the test. He also reports "eye strain" during oculomotor testing.

Clinical Profiles

Nick's primary clinical profile is vestibular, which is supported by his symptoms of dizziness with movement and imbalance, symptom provocation on the VOR and VMS components of the VOMS, follow-up dynamic visual acuity findings, and reported discomfort in busy school environments (see Figure 6.1). His secondary clinical profile is posttraumatic migraine, which is indicated from his reported symptoms of headache, nausea, photosensitivity, and disrupted sleep. In addition, Nick has a tertiary profile of

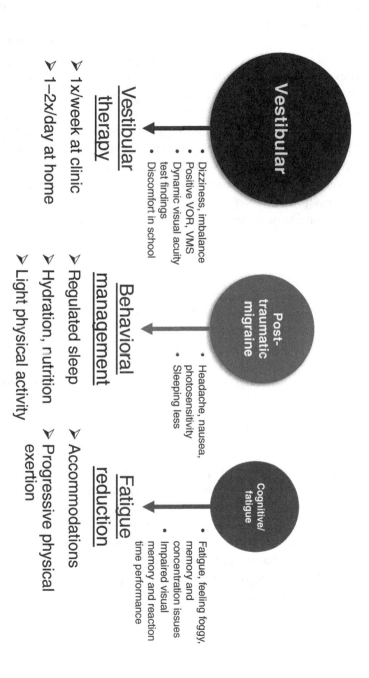

Figure 6.1. Nick's clinical profiles and targeted treatments. VOR = vestibulo-ocular reflex; VMS = visual motion sensitivity.

cognitive-fatigue based on his symptoms of fatigue, feeling foggy, memory and concentration problems, and poor performance on the visual memory and reaction time components of the CNT.

Targeted Treatment Plan

To treat his primary vestibular clinical profile, Nick's vestibular physical therapist prescribes a weekly clinic-based vestibular therapy program together with a home-based program that is performed one to two times each day. Among the exercises included are progressive head movements integrated with motor performance such as turning and catching a ball, walking with head turns, and progressive exposure to busy environments using simulated stimuli in the clinic. To treat the secondary posttraumatic migraine clinical profile, the treating clinical neuropsychologist prescribes an active behavioral management program involving regulated sleep schedule (i.e., 8 hours per night, no napping), and proper hydration and nutrition, and light daily physical activity as tolerated (i.e., 5,000 steps per day). Finally, to treat the tertiary cognitive-fatigue clinical profile, Nick is provided with academic accommodations including breaks throughout the day, additional time between classes, note takers, and additional time for tests and assignments. When his posttraumatic migraine symptoms are under control, he is instructed to begin to increase his physical activity, including dynamic movements, using a prescribed combined aerobic and dynamic exertion program.

Follow-Up/Summary

Nick returns for follow-up appointments 3 and 6 weeks after his concussion. At the 3-week appointment, he reports being compliant with his prescribed treatments and reports overall improvement. He demonstrates improvement in all areas but is still reporting sufficient symptoms and levels of impairment on VOMS and CNT to continue his current prescribed treatments. At the 6-week follow-up, Nick's total PCSS symptom severity score is down to 4, and he is able to complete the VOMS without any symptoms. In addition, his scores on the CNT are back to normal (50th–91st percentile range). At this time, he also successfully completes the aerobic and dynamic Exertional Test components and has no cognitive, vestibular or oculomotor symptoms or impairment after the test.

As a final note to Nick and his family, the clinical neuropsychologist reminds Nick that had he come out of the game right away at the first signs of his concussion, he would have likely cut his recovery time in half and not missed the rest of the season. Nick's case highlights the adverse effects associated with continuing to play through a concussion, especially for younger athletes. In addition, this case emphasizes the importance of a thorough assessment of vestibular function when initial screening tools are positive.

CASE 2. NO PATH TO RECOVERY: THE IMPORTANCE OF SPECIALIZED CARE AFTER CONCUSSION

Initial Presentation

Sheryl is a 40-year-old woman who presents to the clinic approximately 3 months after a concussion. Her chief complaints are "still not feeling right after (her) concussion," intermittent occipital headaches, memory problems, difficulty reading, and concern that her symptoms will affect her ability to perform the duties of her new job. She was initially seen at the emergency department for her concussion, which was the result of a single, direct blow to the back of her head involving a blunt object during an assault and robbery. Her assault occurred late at night, and she was alone when it happened. Immediately after her assault, Sheryl reports wandering for a few minutes before asking for help. The police were then called, and she was transported to the emergency department by Emergency Medical Services. As is often the case, Sheryl did not receive or seek any additional treatment for her concussion beyond an initial diagnosis. She reports concurrent lacerations to her face and the back of her head along with an upper body injury from falling after she briefly lost consciousness from the blow to the head. These injuries had healed completely at the time of presentation.

Injury Information

Sheryl reports being struck in the occipital area of her head by an unknown blunt object and may have hit the frontal aspect of her head during the fall. (Her recollection of the assault and fall is vague.) Results of a CT scan are negative for cerebral bleeding, edema, or other evidence of structural injury. She reports brief (< 30 seconds) loss of consciousness, posttraumatic amnesia for a few hours and considerable confusion and disorientation immediately following her concussion. She also reports experiencing symptoms within the first few hours of her concussion, including frontal and occipital headache, sensitivity to noise, blurry and double vision, trouble focusing and paying attention, and mild nausea.

Medical and Psychosocial History

Sheryl has experienced motion sickness and ocular migraine with aura only since she was in her teens. She also reports being diagnosed with a mood disorder (specifically, bipolar disorder) about 2 years prior to her concussion. She is currently taking lamotrigine and ariprazole and attending biweekly psychotherapy sessions for her bipolar disorder. However, she has remained relatively physically inactive since her injury. In particular, she no longer walks at night following her assault. She also reports current life stressors including starting a new job, financial concerns, and some relationship issues. She has been married to her husband for 4 years.

Clinical Findings

With regard to her current symptoms, Sheryl reports persistent vision problems including bilateral blurred vision with headache and difficulty reading for more than a few minutes at a time; mood disturbance/anxiety including labile affect, being more emotional, and irritable; and being uncomfortable and having headaches and dizziness in busy environments like a park or grocery store. As a result, she is avoidant of these environments and self-protective to avoid any provocation of symptoms. Her daily sleep, nutrition, and hydration are normal. She reports low-level physical activity because she is otherwise occupied and also because she is anxious when feeling symptoms. She expresses concern about potential loss of income because of time away from work as a result of her concussion and about the functional effects of her concussion on her relationships with friends and family. She also reports drinking one to three alcoholic drinks on most days to cope with her symptoms. Sheryl is physically inactive and has become deconditioned. She was unable to complete more than 5 minutes of moderate (65% VO_2 maximum) exertional testing on a stationary cycle.

Her scores on computerized neurocognitive testing indicate mild deficits on visual memory and visual motor processing speed when compared with normative values. Her performances on verbal memory and reaction time are within normal limits. However, she reports symptom provocation (headache, blurry vision) at the conclusion of testing. She performs clinical balance testing without evidence of impairment. However, her NPC distance is 22 centimeters. In addition, results of vestibular and oculomotor screening are highly symptomatic following pursuits and saccades. She is so symptomatic and anxious that she cannot complete the VOR and VMS testing. Results from cervical evaluation are unremarkable.

Referrals and Additional Testing

Sheryl is referred to a behavioral neuro-optometrist and a vestibular physical therapist for additional testing. Her convergence issues are confirmed in subsequent testing by the optometrist, who also notes that she has pronounced nystagmus during pursuit tests. In addition, the optometrist diagnoses her with accommodative insufficiency, which means that the ability of her eye to focus on an object as its distance varies is deficient. The vestibular therapist confirms that Sheryl has positive findings on a dynamic visual acuity test indicating problems with her VOR. However, she tests negative for peripheral vestibular dysfunction, suggesting that her symptoms and impairment are related to central vestibular and oculomotor dysfunction subsequent to the concussion.

Clinical Profiles

Sheryl has a primary oculomotor, secondary vestibular, and tertiary anxiety/mood profiles (see Figure 6.2). The primary oculomotor clinical profile is supported by her very high NPC distance, complaints about reading, and symptom provocation on pursuits and saccades and following computerized neurocognitive testing. Her secondary vestibular profile is supported by her history of motion sickness, inability to perform the VOMS vestibular testing, and discomfort in busy environments. Finally, the tertiary anxiety/mood profile is indicated by her previously diagnosed mood disorder as a risk factor in combination with reported changes in affect, mood, irritability, and emotional response (i.e., potential acute stress disorder), which are also exacerbated by or related to ongoing relationship issues.

Targeted Treatment Plan

Based on Sheryl's primary oculomotor profile, the behavioral neuro-optometrist prescribes a 6-week, home-based, computerized vision therapy program involving specialized goggles and software (see Figure 6.2). To treat Sheryl's vestibular profile, the vestibular physical therapist prescribes a weekly clinic-based vestibular therapy programming together with home-based program that is performed two or three times each day. The tertiary anxiety/mood profile is treated through behavior management and activity. Specifically, the clinical neuropsychologist prescribes an active behavioral management program involving daily physical activity (i.e., 10,000 steps per day), stress management (i.e., deep breathing, mediation), regulated sleep

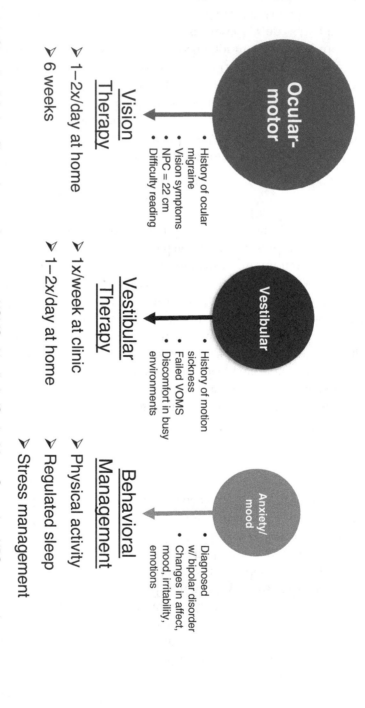

Figure 6.2. Sheryl's clinical profiles and targeted treatments. VOMS = Vestibular/Ocular Motor Screening; NPC = near point convergence; cm = centimeters.

schedule (i.e., 8 hours per night, no napping), and proper hydration and nutrition, including a reduction in alcohol intake to no more than one alcoholic drink per day. Sheryl is also encouraged to seek counseling to deal with her reported (though possibly unrelated) relationship issues, as well as the acute stress of the life-threatening trauma.

Follow-Up/Summary

Sheryl returns 2 weeks after her first appointment—approximately 3½ months following her concussion—and reports good progress and compliance with her prescribed therapies. She also reports less severe symptoms overall. Although she is still having vision-related symptoms, they are less frequent than before, and she is able to read for longer periods of time. However, her NPC distance is still at 12 centimeters, suggesting continued (though improved) impairment. She is able to complete the entire VOMS at this appointment, but she continues to report mild symptom provocation following the saccades and VOR components of the exam. Her scores on computerized neurocognitive testing are now within normal limits, and she is no longer reporting symptom provocation following the test. She reports being much more active (averaging 10,000 steps per day) and drinking less than she had at initial presentation. She is now exposing herself to provocative environments and working through her anxiety and vestibular impairments. She continues to attend her biweekly therapy sessions and to take her prescribed medications for bipolar disorder. She reports feeling better and having a more stable affect. She has also made arrangements to start couples counseling with her husband.

At a 6-week follow-up appointment (approximately 4½ months from her concussion), Sheryl has concluded the vision and vestibular therapy programs and is normal on all clinical findings. In particular, she is able to complete all components of the VOMS without symptom provocation, and her NPC distance is now at 4 centimeters. Perhaps most important to Sheryl, she reports no difficulty reading. Sheryl reports continued increases in physical activity and has recently started kayaking at a local pond near her apartment with a new friend from work. Her mood has stabilized, and she no longer reports any anxiety/mood related symptoms. Sheryl continues to take her anxiety medications and attend biweekly psychotherapy sessions. She also indicated that her new job is going well, and she is no longer drinking other than socially. Sheryl has begun attending weekly couples counseling sessions with her husband and reports an improvement in their relationship.

Sheryl's case highlights the importance of seeking more immediate follow-up care following a concussion. Her oculomotor clinical profile and other profiles could have been treated much earlier and her recovery time lessened significantly had she sought earlier, targeted care for her concussion.

CASE 3. HEADING FOR TROUBLE: LINGERING ANXIETY AFTER CONCUSSION

Initial Presentation

Antonio is a 19-year-old male soccer player who is currently unable to play on his collegiate soccer team because of lingering symptoms following a concussion that he sustained while still in high school approximately 1 year earlier. His primary complaints upon presentation to the clinic include a wide array of symptoms, such as headache, nausea, photosensitivity, dizziness, trouble focusing vision, and fogginess. He also reports disrupted sleep and emotional changes, including irritability, anxiety with panic attack episodes, and overanalyzing things. He has recently taken an official leave of absence from the college in which he was enrolled as a freshman and is currently taking courses at a local community college while living with his parents. He reports being physically inactive (having not played soccer for almost a year), and he has not been very active socially since going to college in the fall.

Injury Information

Antonio's injury occurred during a game in his senior season of high school soccer. He hit his head on the turf following a hard collision with an opponent. He removed himself from the game immediately without any initial symptoms or signs of a concussion. However, within 20 minutes he developed fogginess, dizziness, blurred vision, and trouble focusing visually. His concussion occurred near the end of his senior season, and he did not return to play any more games. However, Antonio intended to continue his playing career at a National Collegiate Athletic Association Division III college near his home. He received initial care from the ATC at his high school and follow-up care from a neurologist, who did not specialize in or typically treat concussion. Results of neuroimaging with computerized tomography (CT) and magnetic resonance imaging (MRI) were normal. Based on the results of a comprehensive neuropsychological evaluation, Antonio was previously prescribed cognitive and physical rest, as well as several medications and supplements, including gabapentin (for headache, sleep), amphetamine/dextroamphetamine (i.e., Adderall, a stimulant for attention, focus, and energy), vitamin B2 (for headache and energy), and magnesium oxide (for headache). He was also referred for cognitive rehabilitation and vision therapy.

Medical and Psychosocial History

The current concussion is Antonio's fifth in 7 years. For each concussion, his symptoms resolved within a week. He has no history of migraine, attention-deficit/hyperactivity disorder (ADHD), learning disorder, or other neurological conditions. Although he reports never having been diagnosed with a psychological disorder, he indicates that he "tends to be anxious," ruminative in his thinking, hypervigilant regarding somatic functioning, and depressed at certain major life events. He also reports that his father has a history of both anxiety and depression and takes medication for ADHD. Academically, Antonio is an excellent (all As) student and wants to major in engineering.

Clinical Findings

Antonio scores a 66 on the PCSS (Lovell & Collins, 1998), which represents a high overall symptom severity score. He endorses 18 of 22 items; his highest rated symptoms (5–6 on a scale up to 6) include headache, sensitivity to light, fatigue, irritability, sadness, feeling more emotional, and visual problems. His CNT scores are all within normal limits (50th–84th percentiles). The results of VOMS screening support symptom provocation (frontal headache and dizziness) following each component of the test. His NPC distance is normal at 1 centimeter. However, an initial cervical screen by a physical therapist reveals tenderness and pain on the left side of the neck with limited range of motion. In addition, Antonio reports increases in headache, dizziness, and nervousness/anxiety following both aerobic and dynamic exertion testing.

Referrals and Additional Testing

As a result of his positive VOMS symptom provocation, Antonio is referred to a vestibular physical therapist for follow-up vestibular testing. The results of his follow-up testing, including Dix Hallpike and supine roll tests, dynamic visual acuity, and gaze stability testing, are negative for BPPV and other vestibular dysfunction. Consequently, central and peripheral vestibular dysfunction are ruled out. Antonio is also referred to a physical medicine and rehabilitation physician for a follow-up cervical examination and X-rays. The results of the X-ray are negative for cervical fracture, but the physician documents limited range of motion and soft tissue pain in the paraspinal and trapezius muscles during the manual physical examination.

Clinical Profiles

Based on the broad and incongruent symptom presentation, high reports of affective symptoms, lack of finding regarding functional impairment, and personal and family history of anxiety and mood issues, Antonio's primary clinical profiles is anxiety/mood (Figure 6.3). However, his broad symptom profile, vestibular symptom provocation, and cervical involvement hint at secondary posttraumatic migraine and tertiary vestibular and cervical clinical profiles.

Targeted Treatment Plan

To treat the anxiety/mood clinical profile, Antonio is prescribed physical activity and instructed to reengage in social activities with family and friends. He is also referred to a psychiatrist with experience treating concussed patients for weekly cognitive behavioral therapy sessions in conjunction with medication management. The posttraumatic migraine clinical profile is addressed using behavioral regulation, including sleep, hydration, nutrition, and progressive exposure to increases in physical exertion. For the vestibular clinical profiles, Antonio is prescribed an initial clinic-based vestibular therapy session along with daily home-based vestibular exercises. To treat Antonio's cervical clinical profile, a combination of physical therapy—including massage and exercises to reduce pain and increase ROM, cyclobenzaprine (a muscle relaxant to treat the neck pain and spasms), and a methylprednisolone dose pack (an oral steroid to reduce inflammation) is indicated. These aspects of Antonio's treatment are provided under the supervision of the physical medicine and rehabilitation physician.

Follow-Up/Summary

Antonio returns for a follow-up appointment 6 weeks after his initial assessment (approximately 1 year and 1½ months following his concussion). At this time, his total PCSS symptom severity score is down to 11, with no single symptoms endorsed above a 2 (mild). He is no longer reporting any symptom provocation following the VOMS items, and his CNT scores are all well above normative values (50th–98th percentile). He is currently taking sertraline, an antidepressant, to enhance his mood; vitamin B2; and magnesium oxide under the supervision of the psychiatrist. He reports attending weekly cognitive behavior therapy sessions with the psychiatrist, which conclude next week with his sixth session, and engaging in normal social activities with friends and family. Antonio has performed well academically in community college and is reapplying to several 4-year colleges to continue his academic studies and begin playing soccer again. From a physical activity perspective, he is training daily—running, resistance training, cycling—and would like to be cleared to start playing soccer again. In addition, he has completed his prescribed vestibular therapy program and is cleared by the

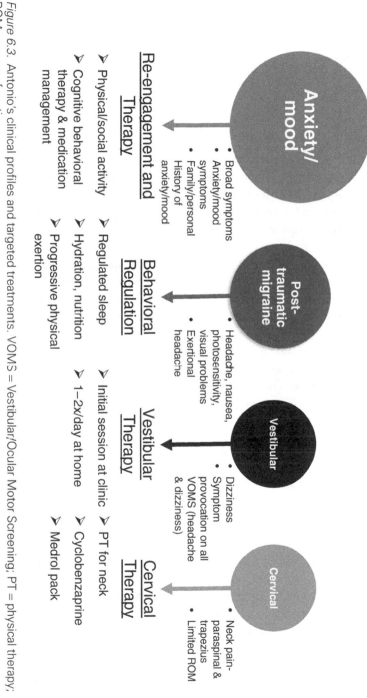

Figure 6.3. Antonio's clinical profiles and targeted treatments. VOMS = Vestibular/Ocular Motor Screening; PT = physical therapy; ROM = range of motion.

vestibular physical therapist following both aerobic and dynamic exertion testing on the Exertional Test. Finally, he reports no neck pain or ROM issues and has discontinued all medications for the pain and inflammation associated with his cervical clinical profile. As a result of the preceding progress, Antonio is cleared for full return to all activities.

This case demonstrates the challenge of disentangling anxiety/mood related issues from other clinical profiles following concussion. In addition, this case emphasizes the importance of a comprehensive assessment and clinical analysis that considers multiple domains, together with follow-up assessments that can inform better diagnosis and more targeted treatment approaches.

CONCLUSION

In the preceding cases, we illustrated the challenges in assessing and treating patients with concussion, including multiple, sometimes overlapping profiles; prioritization of clinical profiles for treatment; and the importance of the role of familial migraine history as a risk factor when assessing ability to play sports. We also highlighted the importance of matching treatments to clinical findings and the multidomain and interdisciplinary perspective that can provide the best outcomes for patients. In so doing, we presented cases that represented three primary profiles commonly seen in our clinic—vestibular, anxiety/mood, and oculomotor—across multiple time points from the few days following a concussion to over a year later. We examined two sport-related concussion cases, as that is what we specialize in at our clinic and because so many concussions that occur are a result of sport and recreational activities. However, we also presented a case involving an assault, which, along with motor vehicle collisions and falls, represents a considerable portion of concussions. In our cases, we included ages ranging from adolescent to adult, and we also looked at both male and female patients. We hope that this chapter helped to bring all of the information from the preceding chapters together to provide a cohesive and real-life look into the clinical profile approach to assessing and treating concussion.

7

AT-RISK POPULATIONS

The information presented in this book is designed to be applicable across different populations and issues related to concussion. However, concussion does not occur in a vacuum; it is influenced by a variety of factors, such as the population affected. Clinicians are likely to experience directly the importance of understanding the unique issues associated with certain populations who are at risk for concussion, including sport participants, youth, and the military. Another group that has received less attention in the literature is underserved populations who may lack access to proper clinical care. It is important for clinicians to understand the nature of these populations to provide the best possible concussion care for them.

Specific issues related to concussion warrant additional discussion. Among the salient issues related to concussion are concerns about repetitive impacts to the head, such as those from heading a soccer ball or playing football, and potential long-term effects, including postconcussion symptoms and chronic traumatic encephalopathy (CTE). The information in this

http://dx.doi.org/10.1037/0000087-008
Concussion: A Clinical Profile Approach to Assessment and Treatment, by A. P. Kontos and M. W. Collins

chapter consolidates information from previous chapters and synthesizes it with additional information to provide easy reference and context for the reader. We begin with a discussion of sport- and recreation-related concussion (SRC).

SPORT AND RECREATION-RELATED CONCUSSION

Much of what we know about concussion from assessment to treatment has emanated from the field of SRC. Although there is information throughout this book from the SRC literature, we think it is important to address a couple of key issues related to SRC. To that end, we address identification, return to play, and concerns related to youth sport, which dovetails into the next section on pediatric concussion.

Identification

One of the main challenges specific to SRC is the early and accurate identification of athletes with suspected concussions. These on-field decisions represent the first line of defense for athletes with potential concussions, because allowing an injured athlete to play can have adverse consequences. However, sport environments involve many potential confounding stressors that may result in symptoms that mimic concussion, making identification particularly challenging. For example, dehydration, fatigue, and excessive heat (which are common consequences of participation in sports) can result in concussion-like symptoms. In addition, factors such as poor sleep and nutrition, including caffeine intake (which is common among athletes), may also foster concussion-like symptoms. Consequently, any initial assessment of concussion in athletes must consider and rule out these potential alternate causes for concussion-like symptoms.

We know that athletes who continue to play while concussed nearly double their recovery time and experience more severe impairments (Elbin, Sufrinko, Schatz, French, Collins, et al., 2016). The athletic trainers and sports medicine professionals who are charged with the task of determining whether an athlete is concussed have limited tools with which to work. Most of the tools to assess this injury focus on signs, symptoms, and brief assessments of cognitive impairment or balance, such as the Sport Concussion Assessment Tool–5 (SCAT-5; Echemendia et al., 2017). Other tools that may be effective in measuring one domain following a concussion, such as oculomotor—like the King-Devick (Galetta et al., 2011)—have been touted by some researchers to be useful in identifying all concussions (e.g., Seidman et al., 2015). However, the evidence does not support this singular approach to identifying concussions.

Recently, the National Football League (NFL) began using an "eye in the sky," an athletic trainer in the press box to identify possible concussions. Although this approach may be useful at elite levels of sport, it is not practical across all levels of sport. Some researchers have proposed developing accelerometer-based biomechanical threshold approaches to help identify concussions (e.g., Rowson et al., 2012). Unfortunately, the simplistic "red light–green light" biomechanical threshold approach to identifying concussion does not seem to be effective and may produce many false positive results. More important, this approach may yield false negative results that result in returning potentially injured athletes to their sport.

In a study we conducted over the course of two ice hockey seasons—involving teams from Pittsburgh, Pennsylvania; Boston, Massachusetts; and Birmingham, Alabama—we found no evidence for a biomechanical threshold to identify concussion (Kontos & Elbin, 2013). Concussions occurred at various linear and rotational accelerations. The accelerometer system we employed used a flashing light on the top of players' helmets to indicate a possible concussion. Unfortunately, this system had the unintended effect of motivating opponents to "light up" other player's helmets! The problem with single sideline assessment approaches, thresholds, and blood biomarkers is that they are predicated on all concussions being alike, which we know is not true. Therefore, until we develop better tools to identify clinical profiles, we must rely on balancing the most comprehensive assessment possible with the limited time frame in which on-field assessments occur to provide the best identification of this injury.

Return to Play

Unlike concussions affecting nonsport participants (with the exceptions of military personnel and individuals with jobs involving physical labor), one of the main concerns regarding sport participants with a concussion is determining when it is safe for them to return to play. For several reasons, return to play is a major concern for clinicians and researchers. The primary reason centers on reducing the likelihood of a second injury to an already injured brain. In addition, return to sport and physical activity, independent of additional injury, may also exacerbate or result in a return of symptoms. Therefore, attempts have been made to standardized return to play protocols (see P. McCrory et al., 2013, 2017). However, these attempts have focused primarily on patient reporting of being symptom free at baseline and following exertion.

Recently, researchers have highlighted the importance of exertion-based approaches to assess readiness to return to play (e.g., Dematteo et al., 2015). We believe that these findings regarding aerobic exertion should be extended to dynamic-based exertion, as discussed in Chapter 4. In addition, expanding postexertion return to play assessments to include cognitive (McGrath et al., 2013) and other assessments such as balance, vestibular, and oculomotor may provide a more complete picture of a patient's readiness for return to play. As we learn more about clinical profiles, researchers and clinicians should reexamine and adjust current return to play approaches to fit each profile and individual patient.

Concerns About Concussions in Youth Sport

Recent estimates suggest that as many as 1.9 million children under 18 years of age have a sport- and recreation-related concussion each year in the United States (Bryan, Rowhani-Rahbar, Comstock, Rivara, & Seattle Sports Concussion Research Collaborative, 2016). Amazingly, the majority (63.5%) of these children do not receive clinical care for their injury (Bryan et al., 2016). This gap between the number of concussions and the number of children receiving appropriate care highlights the importance of not only recognizing concussions in this at-risk age group but also making sure they receive appropriate care. In so doing, we must encourage parents to seek appropriate clinical care for their children with a suspected concussion, especially given the risks of playing while injured (see Chapter 2). This disparity also demonstrates the need to ensure that children have access to appropriate care as well as the insurance coverage to cover that care. In the next section, we discuss the concerns about concussion in pediatric populations that further highlight the importance of concussion in this at-risk population.

CONCUSSION IN PEDIATRIC POPULATIONS: DEVELOPMENTAL CONSIDERATIONS

The pediatric brain is constantly changing, particularly between childhood and adolescence, when behavior, cognitive function, and affect are constantly in flux. Developmental processes in the brain, including myelination, synaptic formation, and pruning, occur through childhood and early adolescence. Specifically, dendritic arborization—growth of neuronal connections—occurs in adolescence (Gogtay et al., 2004). Similarly, synaptic pruning (elimination of rarely used synapses) occurs in late childhood (Paolicelli et al., 2011). Researchers argue that the rapid period of synaptic pruning in adolescence may result in a synaptic vulnerability to brain injury at this time (Giedd, 2004). In addition, many of the neurotransmitters in the pediatric brain, such as glutamate, appear to be more sensitive to brain injury during adolescence (Biagas, Grundl, Kochanek, Schiding, & Nemoto, 1996). A consequence of the preceding processes is an increase in cognitive—though not necessarily behavioral—function during adolescence (Bedard et al., 2002). Consequently, adolescents are much improved over their childhood selves with regard to reaction time, memory, and inhibition (although anyone who has witnessed the behavior of 14-year-olds may have reservations about claims of improved inhibition).

As a result of this dynamic changing landscape of the pediatric brain, it is intuitive to reason that concussive injury to the brain during this time may disrupt any number of these processes. However, in contrast to the linear relationship between age and concussion outcomes suggested in the literature (e.g., Field, Collins, Lovell, & Maroon, 2003; McCrory et al., 2013), it is more likely that vulnerability to the effects of concussion peak in adolescence and then begin to fall off as adolescents move into early adulthood and the brain's development concludes. Recent evidence supports this assertion (e.g., Purcell, Harvey, & Seabrook, 2016). Ultimately, the key question, which has yet to be studied, is whether concussion's effects on the developing brain of pediatric patients are temporary or lasting in nature.

One of the main impediments to assessing concussion in pediatric populations is a lack of age- and developmentally appropriate tools. Recently, pediatric versions of some concussion assessments have been developed. For example, the SCAT-5 (Echemendia et al., 2017) is available in a pediatric version (called the Child SCAT-5; see https://pediatric.impacttest.com/pediatric-concussion/) that covers children between the ages of 5 and 12 years. Similarly, computerized neurocognitive test manufacturers have begun developing pediatric versions of their tests that are appropriate for younger children (e.g., Pediatric ImPACT). Of note, researchers have recently identified a clinical algorithm, the Persistent Post Concussion Symptoms (PPCS) clinical risk score, to identify pediatric patients at risk for long-term (i.e., 28 days) effects from concussion (Zemek et al., 2016). Such an approach may allow clinicians to implement earlier and more effective treatment strategies for these at-risk patients.

With the preceding exceptions, there remains a shortage of developmentally appropriate tools to assess concussion in this age group, leaving clinicians to rely on child/parent symptom reports, which can be unreliable. Gioia (2015) suggested a good approach based on (a) awareness of developmentally appropriate behavior, (b) developmentally appropriate assessments, (c) additional information from parents and other caregivers, and (d) an expectation of a longer recovery for younger children. Based on recent evidence (e.g., Purcell et al., 2016) it is likely that this last tenet should be amended to state "longer recovery in adolescents."

CONCUSSION IN UNDERSERVED POPULATIONS: IMPROVING AWARENESS AND ACCESS TO CARE

Underserved populations include a variety of groups who lack appropriate care for concussion—for example, racial and ethnic minorities as well as individuals living in rural areas with limited access to health care. Previously we reported that groups that are traditionally underserved with regard to concussion management may be at a greater risk for neurocognitive impairment following concussion (Kontos et al., 2010). Researchers have speculated that the greater risk may be due to a lack of access to appropriate care and follow-up treatment (e.g., Bazarian, Pope, McClung, Cheng, & Flesher, 2003). African American youth football players are noted as an example of an underserved group. Researchers have also found that African American children are more likely to have worse clinical outcomes following traumatic brain injury than other ethnic groups (Haider et al., 2007). Previous research speculates that a lack of resources to ensure appropriate care and treatment of concussion and lack of knowledge and awareness about concussion may be leading to this disproportion (e.g., Bazarian et al., 2003; Kontos, Elbin, Covassin, & Larson, 2010).

In response to these findings, we conducted a study in 2012 to examine disparities in concussion awareness, risk, and management for youth in underserved urban areas in Pittsburgh, Pennsylvania (Kontos & Elbin, 2013). A total of 15 administrators and community leaders from seven predominantly African American urban Pittsburgh communities participated in three focus groups to provide insight into concussion in their communities, connect us with community resources, and assist us in the development of a written survey for parents and coaches. The survey focused on concussion awareness, care, knowledge, attitudes, and injury rates. In addition, the survey included hypothetical situations related to concussion outcomes and decision-making. A total of 27 medically diagnosed concussions were reported across the sample. More important, 149 "bell ringers" (i.e., undiagnosed concussions) were reported, suggesting that up to 85% of youth with concussions received no care for their injuries. A total of 109 parents and coaches from across the seven communities completed the survey.

With regard to care, the participants reported that most concussions were treated at the emergency room (65%), whereas only 16% of participants with concussions saw a specialist (Kontos & Elbin, 2013). Most parents of kids with diagnosed concussions reported using University of Pittsburgh Medical Center (UPMC) Children's emergency department for initial care, but they did not typically follow up with a specialist. The results of the study suggest a general lack of on-field management in these communities. Only one community used an appropriately trained sports medicine professional to provide medical coverage, but only during games.

In addition, the participants reported that a lack of insurance and lack of awareness of local clinics for concussion management and treatment were barriers to seeking appropriate care. As part of this project, we also conducted outreach efforts that provided education and awareness to parents and coaches and baseline computerized neurocognitive testing for athletes. Overall, our findings highlight the need for better concussion education/ awareness and access to appropriate clinical care in this at-risk and underserved population.

For rural communities, geographical access to clinical care is a major concern. It is also important to be aware that rural patients with concussion tend to be older and are more likely to have concussions from motor vehicle collisions than their urban counterparts (Stewart, Gilliland, & Fraser, 2014). One of the authors (Anthony Kontos) has worked in rural northern California in Humboldt County for 5 years, and so we know firsthand the challenges of providing concussion education, assessment, and care in rural areas. This massive county of over 4,000 square miles included many Indian reservations (e.g., Hupa, Yurok, Tolowa, Wiyot) and rural communities that were isolated from health care providers. In California, we had the added concern related to a lack of certified athletic trainers in scholastic sports. As a result, emergency medical technicians or school nurses, when available, provided initial concussion care for student athletes, even though they had limited or no training in concussion. Moreover, there were no clinical neuropsychologists or other experts with concussion experience within a 4-hour drive of most patients. As a result, primary care physicians, pediatricians, and urgent care providers with limited or no training in concussion were the primary care providers for patients with concussion.

This limited access to care resulted in our development of the North Coast Concussion Program, which continues to provide concussion education, assessment, and care to student-athletes and community patients in Humboldt County. Our colleague, Justus Ortega, is the current director of this program at Humboldt State University. The program continues to have a substantial impact on concussion care and outcomes in the rural communities in northern California. Moving forward, concussion care in rural areas like Humboldt is likely to be provided through telehealth and other remote access media. In fact, a former postdoctoral fellow at the University of Pittsburgh and current colleague of ours at the University of Arkansas, R. J. Elbin, is working on several concussion telehealth projects to provide concussion awareness, assessment, and care to remote areas of Arkansas. While we believe that telehealth should not replace available in-person care from a clinician trained in concussion, we acknowledge the importance of expanding access to concussion telehealth care options to elevate the standard of care for populations with limited access to care.

CONCUSSION IN THE MILITARY: BLAST CONCUSSIONS AND THE LINK TO POSTTRAUMATIC STRESS DISORDER

More than 370,000 concussions have occurred among U.S. military personnel between 2000 and 2017 (Defense and Veterans Brain Injury Center, 2017). Concussion and other traumatic brain injury have been recognized as the "signature injury" of the wars in Afghanistan and Iraq, with nearly a quarter of deployed military personnel experiencing one or more mild traumatic brain injuries (O'Neil et al., 2013). The related concerns of posttraumatic stress (PTS) symptoms and clinical posttraumatic stress disorder (PTSD) have also garnered considerable attention in military personnel in the past decade. In fact, researchers have noted that PTS and PTSD are more related to concussions and other brain injuries than any other event among military personnel (Belanger et al., 2011). Although concussions in military personnel share many characteristics with concussions in sport- and recreation-related and other civilian populations, several distinct differences are specific to this at-risk population.

Unique Characteristics of Concussion in the Military

Unlike SRCs and concussions in civilian populations, which usually involve blunt direct or indirect forces to the brain, concussion among military personnel may involve a variety of different forces. Concussion in the military can be from blunt, blast, or combined or mixed blast/blunt mechanisms. Blast injury can be further divided into different levels of forces including primary (from blast overpressure), secondary (from flying objects), tertiary (from flying people landing onto objects/ground), and quaternary (from other blast-related injuries). As is evident from these categories of blast injury, most concussions from blast injuries involve many components and are referred to as *mixed* or *combination injuries*. In contrast, pure blast injury, which is less common, involves only primary or blast overpressure forces.

Findings from animal models suggest that the pathophysiology of these pure blast injuries appear to be different from pure blunt injuries and involve functional changes in brain cells (Risling et al., 2011). In contrast, blunt injuries involve a direct mechanical impact to the skull (e.g., blunt weapon; flying debris; violent impact with ground, vehicle, or other structure) that results in linear and rotational forces on the brain. The acceleration/deceleration and rotational forces on the brain from these blunt impacts may cause contusion, axonal shearing, and intracranial bleeding. Blast-blunt combination injuries involve both blunt and one or more blast injury mechanisms. A final unique feature of concussion in military personnel is the importance of return to duty decisions. In sport, return to play decisions may result in subsequent injury, but rarely catastrophic outcomes (second impact syndrome notwithstanding) or harm to others. In contrast, military personnel in both training and combat return to a performance environment with considerable risk. As such, clinical decisions regarding return to duty among military personnel should err on the side of caution.

The Link Between Posttraumatic Stress Disorder and Concussion

In military populations, concussions and more severe traumatic brain injury have been linked with PTS and PTSD (Hoge et al., 2008). It is estimated that PTS symptoms are reported acutely by approximately 40% of U.S. military personnel following exposure to concussion (Hoge et al., 2008). Researchers have reported that 42% of recent U.S. military veterans with a concussion history report concurrent PTS symptoms (Lew et al., 2008). In our research with U.S. Army Special Operations Forces, we found that PTS symptoms were reported in 28% of personnel (Kontos, Kotwal, et al., 2013). This is particularly surprising because these personnel are selected for resiliency and are less likely to report symptoms in the first place. More important, we reported a link between concussion history and residual symptoms of PTS. Specifically, personnel with a history of blunt concussions were 3.6 times more likely to report clinical PTS symptoms than personnel with no history (Kontos, Kotwal, et al., 2013).

Not surprisingly, personnel with blast (4.2 times) and blast/blunt combination (5.4 times) were even more likely to report clinical PTS symptoms than were those with no history of concussion. We also found support for a dose–response gradient for exposure to blast and residual PTS symptoms. In fact, personnel with exposure to three or more concussions from blast or blast/blunt combination forces were twice as likely to report clinical PTS symptoms as those with exposure to only one blast concussion (Kontos, Kotwal, et al., 2013). These findings draw attention to the unique concern and potential effects associated with repeated blast-related concussions and chronic lower level exposure to blast among military personnel.

Repeated Exposure to Blast Impacts

Similar to concerns about repeated exposures from boxing, playing football, or heading a soccer ball among athletes, repeated exposure to blast impacts among military personnel pose health concerns. Two separate but related concerns are relevant in this context: repeated blast exposures that result in concussions, and repeated blast exposures that are subclinical or lower level in nature. The former, while problematic, are more overt and likely to result in appropriate clinical care. In contrast, asymptomatic low-level blast exposures are more insidious, and therefore, less likely to result in clinical care or assessment until symptoms and impairment are evident. In our research with U.S. Army Special Operations Forces, we have seen personnel with up to nine diagnosed blast-related concussions (Kontos, Kotwal, et al., 2013). Suffice it to say, these individuals have substantial residual symptoms and cognitive impairment.

In a recent study we conducted in this population, we found evidence that a history of even a single blast concussion is related to worse impairment and symptoms following a subsequent concussion (Kontos et al., 2015). However, we know next to nothing about the effects of exposure to low-level blast forces (e.g., those with exposures to explosive breach and heavy munitions) on military personnel. In one of the few studies on low-level blast exposure in military personnel, Tate and colleagues (2013) reported that New Zealand military personnel with the highest biomarker scores (i.e., evidence of brain perturbation) following breacher training scored worse on neurocognitive tests and reported more symptoms. Similarly, Carr et al. (2015) found a relationship between low-level blast exposure and cognitive impairment in a small sample ($n = 10$) of breacher instructors from the U.S. Marine Corps. Although these studies suggest that exposure to low-level blast forces may result in both symptoms and impairment, the findings are tentative and require further replication in larger samples and longer term follow-up assessments. Many law enforcement officers also have chronic exposure to blast forces from breacher training and duty and warrant attention from researchers and clinicians. Therefore, clinicians should be aware of military and law enforcement patients' occupational exposure to blast and consider that exposure in assessing risk, prognosis, and treatment for these patients.

Surging Veteran Population and Concussions in Training

Many recent military personnel who served in wars in Afghanistan and Iraq and the ongoing war on terrorism are now transitioning to civilian life and medical care in the Veterans Affairs (VA) system. However, the VA health care system is currently not prepared to handle the influx of patients with concussion, PTS, and related issues. Moreover, civilian clinicians who treat former military personnel often lack sufficient insight into and experience with the specific issues surrounding concussion in this population as outlined earlier. As a result, there is a gap in the available concussion and related care for recently discharged military personnel. Moving forward, we must address this gap in order to avoid the consequences of mismanaged care for this injury.

One final note: Concussion, PTS, and other brain injury related issues do not occur only in theater or during combat missions; many concussions occur during training (e.g., ordnance, breaching), sports/recreational activities, and from motor vehicle collisions both on and off base. As such, we hope that research on concussion, PTS, and other related issues that affect military personnel continue to attract funding, even as combat exposure declines.

REPETITIVE IMPACTS TO THE HEAD

Soccer Heading

Soccer is unique among sports because it is the only sport that involves purposeful use of the head to control, pass, or shoot the ball. This action of soccer heading has drawn considerable attention from policymakers, clinicians, researchers, parents, coaches, and athletes for its potential effects on the brain, particularly among younger players. In fact, in response to a recent lawsuit and to minimize concussions from heading in youth soccer, U.S. Soccer enacted guidelines restricting heading completely under age 11 and limiting it for players aged 11 to 13 years. However, these guidelines and much of the speculation for the negative effects of soccer heading are not supported by empirical evidence.

Research on the effects of soccer heading on the brain can trace its roots to the 1970s and 1980s through the early 1990s, when a series of studies of former professional soccer players from Scandinavia suggested a link between heading and impairment later in life (e.g., Tysvaer & Løchen, 1991; Tysvaer & Storli, 1981). Although these studies started the ball rolling in this line of inquiry, they were wrought with methodological flaws (e.g., use of retrospective soccer heading data based on player recall) and did not consider factors such as concussion history in their findings. Nonetheless, these studies prompted additional, more well-controlled research from the 1990s through the present (e.g., Matser et al., 1998; Putukian et al., 2000). However, overall, these studies have provided largely equivocal findings regarding the effects of heading on impairment, symptoms, and other concussion-related outcomes.

In a study on the effects of soccer heading in elite youth players, we found no association between reported soccer heading exposure and cognitive impairment or concussion-related symptoms (Kontos, Dolese, Elbin, Covassin, & Warren, 2011). Our results echo those of other researchers who reported no negative effects related to exposure to soccer heading (Dorminy et al., 2015; Kaminski, Cousino, & Glutting, 2008). However, some researchers have reported a relationship between acute and long-term soccer heading exposure and adverse outcomes (e.g., Haran, Tierney, Wright, Keshner, & Silter, 2013; M. R. Zhang, Red, Lin, Patel, & Sereno, 2013). A variety of factors. such as quantifying heading exposure, measure of impairment and symptoms, and study design, may account for the difference among studies.

To explore these inconsistent findings, we recently concluded a meta-analytic review of the soccer heading literature and found no support for an overall effect of heading across studies (Kontos, Braithwaite, et al., 2017). However, the results of our analysis suggested that any effects are subtle and likely limited to professional players who had substantial long-term exposure to heading. Our results were in line with a previous systematic review conducted by Maher, Hutchison, Cusimano, Comper, and Schweizer (2014), which also indicated no relationship between soccer heading and any negative consequences. Regardless of these empirical findings to the contrary, concerns remain among parents, coaches, athletes, and the media about soccer heading.

Not surprisingly, the concerns about soccer heading from parents, coaches, and athletes, together with the constant focus on heading the ball in the media, have led manufacturers to develop products aimed at minimizing the impacts from soccer heading. While these products may be useful at reducing the likelihood of lacerations to the scalp, their effect on reducing impacts to the brain from heading the ball are not supported by independent research. We conducted a small, randomized trial of the effects of soccer headgear on impairment and symptoms following a bout of soccer heading (Elbin, Beatty, et al., 2015). Our findings indicated that there were no protective effects for the protective soccer headgear (a soft, headband-type head gear) that we tested. In contrast, we actually found that players who were randomly assigned to wearing the protective headgear performed worse on some cognitive tests following a bout of soccer headers. This finding, though tentative and with only a small sample size, highlights the potential unintended effect of wearing protective headgear in sports like soccer that do not traditionally involved such equipment; those who wore protective head gear engaged in more aggressive behaviors, thereby increasing their exposure to heading and risk from potential concussions caused by collisions while heading the ball.

American Football

In American football, where protective headgear has been an integral part of safety equipment since the early 1900s, there is also concern regarding the potential effects of repetitive subconcussive blows to the head. More specifically, there is concern about repetitive subconcussive blows from playing American football, especially for players in certain positions. At a recent Safety in College Football summit we attended, it was suggested that certain positions, such as offensive and defensive lineman in particular, might have higher exposure to impacts involving the head (A. Kontos, personal communication, February 10, 2016). Researchers have begun to investigate these concerns by using accelerometers to measure rotational and linear head accelerations (e.g., Broglio, Eckner, et al., 2011), and then relating the total amount of accelerations in g's or rads/s^2 and number of "impacts" or frequency of accelerations above a certain limit. These studies focus on season-based or practice-based cumulative exposure in relation to acute/immediate or postseason symptoms and impairment.

Findings thus far offer limited or no evidence for a link between playing American football at youth, high school, or collegiate levels and acute adverse effects (e.g., McCaffrey, Mihalik, Crowell, Shields, & Guskiewicz, 2007; Munce, Dorman, Thompson, Valentine, & Bergeron, 2015). Interestingly, although youth players experienced similar levels of head accelerations to high school and collegiate players, they did not experience any adverse acute effects from these exposures (Munce et al., 2015). Other researchers have suggested that there is also no link between cumulative exposure to impacts to the head and concussion risk (Eckner, Sabin, Kutcher, & Broglio, 2011). Despite this lack of evidence, researchers have demonstrated that limiting full contact practices can reduce head impacts in high school players (Broglio, Williams, O'Connor, & Goldstick, 2016).

Other researchers have focused on the chronic effects of exposure to American football and symptoms and impairment. Recent findings by Montenigro et al. (2017) suggest that cumulative exposure to head impacts in 93 former high school and collegiate American football players was associated with depression and cognitive impairment. Similarly, Stamm and colleagues (2015) reported that earlier exposure to American football was related to cognitive impairment among former NFL players. However, this study and others like it have used retrospective methods, which are confounded by cohort and selection effects and other factors (e.g., learning disability, mental health, substance abuse). In a study of retired NFL players, Solomon and colleagues (2016) found no relationship between exposure to youth football and neurological or neuroradiological findings. In conclusion, while additional prospective/longitudinal research in this area is needed, particularly in youth football, there is limited and somewhat equivocal evidence for the role of cumulative subconcussive impacts to the brain from playing American football on impairment and symptoms. However, the long-term effects of repeated concussive impacts are less clear.

Chronic Traumatic Encephalopathy

One of the most controversial issues related to concussion is CTE (previously referred to as *pugilistic dementia*, *punch drunk*, and *boxer's brain*), a form of neurodegeneration thought to be the result of an accumulation of hyperphosphorylated tau protein in the brain. At present, CTE can be diagnosed only upon death and a concomitant autopsy of brain tissue.

Whereas there is fairly consistent agreement among pathologists on the neuropathological characteristics of CTE (McKee et al., 2016), there is less agreement on the causes and clinical manifestation of CTE. The clinical hallmarks of CTE include irritability, depression, cognitive impairment, motor problems, and other concussion-like symptoms (Montenigro, Bernick, & Cantu, 2015). Although the concept of CTE is not new—as Solomon and Sills (2014) pointed out in their review, CTE was originally described over 85 years ago—its rediscovery and the coinciding media spotlight on concussion in sports like American football and in the military together have combined to intensify interest in CTE. As a result, the public and media are under the impression that evidence for CTE is strong because of what Solomon and Sills referred to as the *availability cascade*, where the majority of focus is on positive results for CTE and its proposed link to sports and concussion. Interest in this condition was further stoked by a relatively short article and accompanying movie titled *Concussion*, which focused on the travails of the rediscovery of CTE by Bennett Omalu. Consequently, CTE is frequently in the news, and its link to sports and concussion is assumed to be fact.

We believe it is important for clinicians, the media, and the public to discuss and debate the issue of CTE, but we think it is even more important for researchers to conduct sound methodological studies on CTE and for clinicians to have sound discussions with their patients, patients' parents, and others about CTE. As Love and Solomon (2015) suggested, we need to have an evidence-based discussion to separate fact from hype. To date, the majority of what is known about CTE comes from a handful of case studies and case series of former athletes and military personnel with pathologically diagnosed evidence of CTE (e.g., McKee et al., 2009; Omalu, Hamilton, Kamboh, DeKosky, & Bailes, 2010). In addition, there is evidence that not all neurological deficits associated with multiple concussions and a career in the NFL have pathological evidence of hyperphosphorylated tau, suggesting an alternate mechanism for neurodegeneration (Hazrati et al., 2013). In summary, current evidence suggests that some individuals may develop a chronic form of neurodegeneration that is correlated to hyperphosphorylated tau protein in the brain in some, but not all cases.

We also do not definitively know what causes CTE, nor do we know if it is caused by concussions or subconcussive impacts. In fact, there is no causal evidence for a link between concussion and CTE (Davis, Castellani, & McCrory, 2015). As Iverson, Gardner, McCrory, Zafonte, and Castellani (2015) pointed out, the clinical features of CTE may be related to age, depression, and other neurodegenerative processes. We do not even know the prevalence of CTE in at-risk populations or the general population.

What we do know is that we need additional research on the epidemiology and etiology of CTE to determine its prevalence in at-risk and the general population, as well as risk factors for the development of CTE. Until then, we believe that we should temper the fear associated with CTE until we have more empirical evidence to support or refute current hypotheses. As Solomon and Sills (2014) suggested, we need to let the empirical evidence catch up to the media and public perception of CTE. We encourage readers to examine the extant literature on CTE for themselves. We also urge clinicians to inform patients about the state of the science regarding CTE and to help dispel the fears associated with this poorly understood phenomenon.

CONCLUSION

Concussions can affect anyone in nearly any activity. However, sports and recreation, pediatric, underserved, and military personnel populations are particularly at risk. SRC presents several challenges to clinicians, ranging from identification of the injury to determination of safe return to play. Given that the pediatric brain, particularly during adolescence, may be at increased risk from the effects of concussion, additional emphasis on this population from both a research and clinical perspective is warranted. With regard to underserved individuals, improving awareness and education about concussion together with enhancing access to community-based clinical care are paramount. Telehealth care for concussion may offer solutions to reach remote, rural underserved populations.

Although there is slightly less visibility and emphasis on the effects of concussion in the military as the recent wars in Afghanistan and Iraq have receded into the background, the lingering effects of previous concussions and the continued risk of injury from training highlight the need to continue efforts at better understanding and treating concussion in military personnel. In particular, repetitive military training that involves exposure to blast forces such as breacher and munitions-related blasts needs to be better understood, identified earlier, and treated appropriately. In addition, understanding and extricating PTSD from the effects of concussion is critical to inform better and more targeted treatments for active duty military personnel and veterans. Finally, the issue of CTE and other potential long-term neurodegenerative effects that are proposed to be related to concussions or repeated impacts to the head require more empirical evidence using prospective and longitudinal methodologies.

8

CONCUSSION MOVING FORWARD: WHAT'S NEXT?

The field of concussion has evolved dramatically over the previous decade and even more so compared with the decade before that. Advances in assessment, treatment, and understanding of risk factors, combined with increased awareness, have changed considerably what we know and how we care for patients with concussion. Most important, concussion is now viewed as a treatable injury, not something simply to be managed. However, the field of concussion continues to evolve at a rapid pace and will continue to do so for the foreseeable future. As indicated in previous chapters, advances in treatment, exertion-based approaches, and emerging neuroimaging and blood biomarkers assessments represent a handful of changes currently moving the field of concussion. With this rapidly changing environment in mind, we conclude with a brief review of the areas in which change is most imminent or needed.

http://dx.doi.org/10.1037/0000087-009
Concussion: A Clinical Profile Approach to Assessment and Treatment, by A. P. Kontos and M. W. Collins

CHANGING THE PARADIGM FOR CONCEPTUALIZING AND TREATING CONCUSSION

On October 15–16, 2015, we convened the Targeted Evaluation and Active Management (TEAM) Approaches to Concussion meeting in Pittsburgh, Pennsylvania. This meeting included 40 experts on concussion from across the United States as well as more than 20 invited participants from a variety of public health (e.g., Centers for Disease Control and Prevention [CDC], National Institutes of Health [NIH], OneMind) sport (e.g., US Soccer, USA Football, USA Rugby), and military (Defense and Veterans Brain Injury Center, U.S. Army Materiel Research and Medical Command) organizations. The purpose of this meeting, which was supported by grants from the National Football League and UPMC, was to discuss the current status of concussion treatments and new approaches to conceptualizing and treating this injury. In the process, we hoped to come to some agreement on specific statements and then develop a white paper to disseminate this information to other professionals and the public. In short, we wanted to recognize where we were as a field and focus on changing the paradigm for how we think about and treat concussion. The meeting was much needed and long overdue. As one might imagine, the undertaking of such a task was daunting to say the least. One participant likened the process to herding a bunch of cats.

It was therefore to our pleasant surprise when we walked out of the final day's meetings with majority agreement on 16 key statements and several future directions related to treating concussion (see Exhibit 8.1). In particular, we agreed that "concussion is treatable" and that "concussions are characterized by diverse symptoms and impairments resulting in different clinical profiles and recovery trajectories" (M. W. Collins et al., 2016). These agreements substantiate the notion that the heterogeneity of concussion necessitates the use of evolving clinical profiles and that treatments for this injury should be active and targeted to specific profiles. Although the 2016 Concussion in Sport Group Berlin Consensus Statement uses the more active term *treatment* instead of the more passive term *management* when discussing clinical care for concussion, it does not mention much in the way of specific types of treatment or targeted approaches beyond focusing on specific symptoms (P. McCrory et al., 2017). In addition, the Berlin consensus documents still emphasize an initial period of rest despite growing evidence to the contrary for many patients and clinical profiles, and as such, do not really emphasize active treatments for this injury. In contrast, the agreements from the Pittsburgh treatment meeting lend much-needed support to the conceptual approach involving clinical profiles and an active, targeted approach to treatment as discussed in Chapters 1 and 5, this volume. We hope clinics across North America and beyond will adopt this approach.

EXHIBIT 8.1
The 16 Statements of Agreement

Summary of the Current Approach to Treating Concussion
1. Prior expert consensus for management of concussion included a) no same-day return to play, b) prescribed physical and cognitive rest until asymptomatic, c) accommodations at school/work as needed, and d) progressive aerobic exertion-based return to play based on symptoms.
2. Previous consensus statements have provided limited guidance with regard to the active treatment of concussion.
3. There is limited empirical evidence for the effectiveness of prescribed physical and cognitive rest and no multisite randomized clinical trial for prescribed rest following concussion.
4. Prescribed physical and cognitive rest may not be an effective strategy for all patients following concussion.
5. Strict brain rest (e.g., stimulus deprivation, "cocoon" therapy) is not indicated and may have detrimental effects on patients following concussion.
6. Although most individuals follow a rapid course of recovery over several days to weeks following injury, concussions may involve varying lengths of recovery.
7. Recovery from concussion is influenced by modifying factors, the severity of injury, and the type and timing of treatment that is applied.

Heterogeneity and Evolving Clinical Profiles of Concussion
8. Concussions are characterized by diverse symptoms and impairments in function resulting in different clinical profiles and recovery trajectories.
9. Thorough multidomain assessment is warranted to properly evaluate the clinical profiles of concussion.
10. A multidisciplinary treatment team offers the most comprehensive approach to treating the clinical profiles associated with concussion.

Targeted Evaluation and Active Management Approach to Concussion: Specific Strategies
11. Concussion is treatable.
12. Preliminary evidence suggests that active rehabilitation may improve symptom recovery more than prescribed rest alone after concussion.
13. Active treatment strategies may be initiated early in recovery following concussion.
14. Matching targeted and active treatments to clinical profiles may improve recovery trajectories following concussion.
15. Patients returning to school/work while recovering from concussion benefit from individualized management strategies.
16. Pharmacological therapy may be indicated in selected circumstances to treat certain symptoms and impairments related to concussion.

Note. From "Statements of Agreement From the Targeted Evaluation and Active Management (TEAM) Approaches to Treating Concussion Meeting Held in Pittsburgh, October 15–16, 2015," by M. W. Collins, A. P. Kontos, D. O. Okonkwo, J. Almquist, J. Bailes, M. Barisa, . . . R. Zafonte, 2016, *Neurosurgery, 79,* pp. 912–929. Copyright 2016 by Oxford University Press. Adapted with permission.

RECOGNIZING THAT CONCUSSION IS TREATABLE

Passive concussion "management" strategies are fading quickly. Although prescribed rest is still a viable acute intervention for some patients, targeted, active treatments involving exertion, vestibular, vision, and other therapies offer a more effective approach for patients with certain clinical profiles (see Chapter 5). We recently summarized statements of agreement for treating patients with concussion that provides traction to an active approach (M. W. Collins et al., 2016). As treatment paradigms evolve, we need empirical data on the timing and dosage resulting in the best clinical outcomes. In so doing, we can determine which treatments best match clinical profiles and facilitate and accelerate a more complete recovery for patients. Although evidence-based dose response approaches to therapy are futuristic, these approaches are worthwhile goals in concussion treatment.

EXPANDING THE ROLE OF EXERTION
IN TREATING CONCUSSION

Physical and mental activity improves our well-being. Recent evidence suggests that physical activity promotes neurogenesis (DiFeo & Shors, 2017) and overall mental health (Carter, Morres, Meade, & Callaghan, 2016). We employ active, physical exertion–based approaches to treat concussion as part of regular patient care. However, the evidence for physical exertion as an active treatment is only now coming to light (Dematteo et al., 2015; Leddy et al., 2010). In contrast, although physical activity may increase transient symptoms (Silverberg et al., 2016), little is known about the effects of cognitive activity on patients following concussion. Questions remain concerning the timing, frequency, and intensity of exertion and whether cognitive and physical exertion should be combined or used and researched independently. In any case, it is apparent that exertion will play a growing role in our concussion treatment approach and may one day be included in the "standard of care" approach.

USING NEUROIMAGING AND BLOOD BIOMARKERS
TO ASSESS CONCUSSION

Undoubtedly, objective neuroimaging and blood biomarkers are needed to augment current clinically based approaches to assessing and monitoring recovery from concussion. While considerable advances have been made during the past decade in neuroimaging involving diffusion tensor imaging, high-definition fiber tracking, functional near-infrared spectroscopy, electroencephalography, and other modalities, no clinically accepted neuroimaging protocol for patients with concussion yet exists. Moreover, the evidence for neuroimaging is inconsistent (see Chapter 4), and advances are further complicated by company-specific imaging sequences and incompatible systems. Despite these challenges, several efforts are currently underway to accelerate and standardize approaches to imaging the brain of concussed patients. In fact, several multisite clinical neuroimaging studies to identify and track recovery from concussion are ongoing at the University of Pittsburgh. Current approaches to blood biomarker research have been characterized by inconsistent findings and used single, proprietary biomarker assessments developed by companies with a vested interest in the outcome. Research on biomarkers must be agnostic and focus on the best combination of markers for each clinical profile. The success of neuroimaging and blood biomarkers is contingent upon a clinical profile informed by assay-based approaches to assessing concussion (see Chapter 4).

USING RANDOMIZED CONTROLLED TRIALS OF TARGETED TREATMENTS FOR CONCUSSION

Unquestionably, we need randomized controlled trials (RCTs) in sufficiently large populations to determine the true effectiveness of interventions for patients with concussion. To accomplish this, a shift in funding toward clinical trials is vital. Leveraging both the resources and scales of existing studies such as the National Collegiate Athletic Association–Department of Defense, TRACK TBI, and TEAM TBI projects will jumpstart the process of evaluating concussion treatments. A smart approach when designing and evaluating the success of RCTs for concussion is essential. Additionally, a movement toward conducting targeted trials with focus on treating specific clinical profiles and differentiating treatment effects within studies to determine specific treatment effects is necessary to define concussion treatment. Finally, clinicians and researchers need to be flexible and open to new approaches and willing to randomly assign patients to less effective treatments in order to substantiate effective approaches through empirical evidence. In the meantime, researchers and clinicians shall continue examining the role of specific treatments using case and case series approaches. As trends from these initial research steps emerge, we must move to observational trials that assess the comparative efficacies of treatment modalities for specific clinical profiles. Efforts to assess targeted treatment effectiveness without regard to clinical profile are likely to fail.

INCREASING OUTREACH AND AWARENESS
TO CHANGE BEHAVIORS

"Awareness followed by action" should be the mantra for all education/ awareness efforts for concussion moving forward. Education efforts should be framed on evidence-based information and target broad audiences. However, a balance must be sought so that these efforts do not create unnecessary fear about concussion such that normal sports-play and activity are hindered. Ongoing efforts, including the CDC Heads Up and Heads up Pittsburgh efforts (see Chapters 4 and 5), provide good starting points from which evidence-based concussion awareness can be built to maximize awareness and minimize fear.

Moving forward, education efforts must use behavior change models that have proven successful in other health-related behaviors, such as smoking cessation and physical activity. To this end, the National Collegiate Athletic Association (NCAA) and CDC have aimed to change behaviors related to concussion (i.e., reporting of concussion, seeking care following an injury). Hopefully, additional funds will be available to continue concussion awareness strategy research; fear-based strategies and hyperawareness of injury risk should be avoided. Concussion education efforts should extend beyond sport to include military and pediatric populations. Because a majority (56%) of children with concussion never seek clinical care (O'Kane et al., 2014), secondary prevention focused on recognizing the signs and symptoms of concussion and seeking appropriate care is needed. Doing so will limit significantly the morbidity from protracted symptoms, impairment, and recovery from untreated concussions.

DEVELOPING EVIDENCE-DRIVEN GUIDELINES

Creating policies to prevent concussion and concussion effects in pediatric, sport, military, and the general population are overall goals. These policy goals have good intentions, but they must be driven by evidence. The recent US Soccer heading guidelines, enacted in response to a lawsuit settlement and based on expert opinion rather than evidence, represent an approach in which intentions were good, but the outcome was not based on evidence. Reactively setting arbitrary age cutoffs and developing guidelines based on expert opinion and testimony have no place in concussion research and awareness. Instead, building empirical evidence through sound methodological studies that inform sensible guidelines to improve the safety of at-risk populations will be the standard. The NCAA Safety in Football and Inter-Association Concussion Guidelines (NCAA Sport Science Institute, 2016) are good examples of evidence-based guidelines that use empirical data to substantiate policy, rule changes, and clinical care decision-making.

USING METADATA AND DEVELOPING COMMON DATA ELEMENTS THAT ARE SPECIFIC TO CONCUSSION

One of the biggest challenges in concussion research is aggregating data across studies using metadata and meta-analytic methods. Because of publication bias toward repeated studies, current one-off studies are rarely replicated. Although individual empirical studies are important and add to our understanding of this injury, trends across multiple studies, sites, and populations foster evidence for change in the field and patient treatment. To this end, the NIH, U.S. Department of Defense (DoD), and other agencies developed and support the Federal Interagency Traumatic Brain Injury Research (FITBIR) informatics system. The goal of this system is to provide a vehicle in which researchers can aggregate data across studies using common data elements (CDEs) specific to traumatic brain injury (TBI). Although this effort is well intended, it uses TBI-specific CDEs, which have limited application and use in the field of concussion. In short, concussion-specific CDEs allow for better communication and analysis across studies.

In response to the need for concussion-specific CDEs, in 2017, the National Institute of Neurological Disorders and Stroke (NINDS) published CDEs for sport- and recreation-related concussion. These CDEs cover acute, subacute, and chronic postinjury time periods and involved input from 34 experts in sport-related concussion. The goals of the CDE process were to develop core, supplemental highly recommended, and supplemental measures across each injury time period that would inform future research in concussion. Anthony Kontos served as chair for the subacute working group of the NINDS CDEs, with Steven Broglio as chair for the acute and Lisa Wilde and Kathryn Schneider as co-chairs for the chronic group. The National Institute of Neurological Disorders and Stroke (n.d.) CDEs for sport concussion and efforts like FITBIR permit a better understanding of concussion and promote more effective and comparable communication of findings across studies and different disciplines.

THE CHANGING LANDSCAPE OF CONCUSSION

We often joke that now is both the best and worst time to be involved in concussion. It is the best time because we know more about this injury now than ever before and we keep learning more with each passing day. There is also a greater emphasis on funding for research on concussion from federal (e.g., NIH, DoD), foundation, and corporate sources, and peer-reviewed articles on concussion appear in many medical and psychological journals on a regular basis (see Exhibit 8.2). In 2015, several concussion-specific journals, including *Current Research: Concussion* and *Concussion*, went into circulation.

EXHIBIT 8.2
Major Sources of Funding and Peer-Reviewed Publications
That Support Concussion Research

Major sources of funding for concussion research	Peer-reviewed journals that include articles on concussion
Department of Defense	*American Journal of Sports Medicine*
National Collegiate Athletic Association	*Archive of Clinical Neuropsychology*
	Brain Imaging and Behavior
National Football League	*Clinical Journal of Sports Medicine*
National Institutes of Health (including National Institute of Neurological Disorders and Stroke; National Institute on Deafness and Other Communication Disorders; and Eunice Kennedy Shriver National Institute of Child Health and Human Development)	*Journal of American Medical Association (JAMA)*
	JAMA-Pediatrics
	Journal of Athletic Training
	Journal of Neurotrauma
	Journal of Neurology, Neurosurgery and Medicine & Science in Sports & Exercise
	New England Journal of Medicine
National Operating Committee of Standards for Athletic Equipment	*Psychiatry*
	Journal of Pediatrics
Veterans Affairs	*NeuroImage*
	Neuropsychology
	Neurosurgery
	Pediatrics

Information about concussion is also readily accessible to the general population, with stories appearing in nearly every newspaper and sports magazine and on countless websites. In fact, entire Internet blogs focus on concussion (e.g., The Concussion Blog). However, the rapidly changing landscape of concussion has also resulted in a lot of misinformation and misconception about this injury both in the media and general public, as well as among many clinicians and researchers. In addition, a lot of individuals and companies have jumped on the concussion bandwagon to make money and a name for themselves by offering everything from equipment to prevent concussion and concussion diagnostic tests to treatments that can "cure" concussions. As a result, it is more and more difficult to discern the fact from the fiction surrounding this injury. In the sections that follow, we present a brief review of some of the positive and negative developments resulting from the evolving concussion landscape.

COUNTERING FEAR WITH FACTS

Science and evidence-based information regarding concussion represents a collective whisper buried in the cacophony of sensationalized anecdotes, exaggerated claims, and hyperbolic media attention for misinformation.

As our recently commissioned Harris Poll indicated, 25% of parents prevent their children from playing sports because of concerns about concussions (M. Collins, 2015). To counter this omnipresent fear and misinformation, expansion of public health efforts providing evidence-based information about concussion is compulsory. Efforts such as the ReThink Concussion campaign for parents and patients (UPMC Sports Medicine Concussion Program, 2017), the American Psychological Association (n.d.) Concussion Toolkit for psychologists, and the CDC (2017) Heads Up Concussion program for clinicians, parents, and athletes must continually be supported and expanded. Most of these efforts target sport populations, but some efforts, such as the American Psychological Association Concussion Toolkit, include military and civilian populations. Moving forward, expanding these efforts will include other at-risk groups, including pediatric, older adult, and underserved populations.

EXPANDING THE PROFESSIONAL INTERDISCIPLINARY SUBSPECIALTY OF CONCUSSION RESEARCH AND CLINICAL CARE

The growth of research and clinical care for concussion has been mirrored by expanded programming at psychology and other conferences, as well as the development of subspecialty conferences and professional groups focused on concussion. Professional organizations, including the American Psychological Association, the American College of Sports Medicine, the National Academy of Neuropsychology, the International Neuropsychology Society, and the National Athletic Trainers Association, now regularly include concussion-focused continuing education and research programming in their conferences. However, experts in concussion are coming together more frequently to conduct stand-alone conferences focused solely on concussion. For example, in 2013, the University of Pittsburgh Medical Center's Sports Medicine Concussion Program hosted the Emerging Frontiers in Concussion conference in downtown Pittsburgh. More than 450 professionals representing a variety of health professions attended.

Some professionals have come together to form concussion-related subspecialty professional organizations. In 2013, the first meeting of the Sport Neuropsychology Society was held in Minneapolis, Minnesota. This group's focus is on establishing and promoting the growing field of sport neuropsychology, with a primary emphasis on concussion. The Sport Neuropsychology Society represents an outgrowth of the broader field of clinical neuropsychology, with many of its members and much of its conference programming focusing on sport-related concussion. More recently, American Academy

International and National Professional Organizations that Focus
on Concussion Research or Clinical Care

Academy of Orthopaedic Society for Sports Medicine
American Academy of Family Physicians
American Academy of Neurology: Sport Neurology group
American Academy of Neurological Surgeons
American Academy of Pediatrics
American College of Sports Medicine
American Medical Society for Sports Medicine
American Psychological Association: Divisions 19 (Society for Military Psychology),
    22 (Rehabilitation Psychology), 40 (Society for Clinical Neuropsychology), and
    47 (Society for Sport, Exercise & Performance Psychology)
Association of Applied Sport Psychology
Brain Injury Association of America
International Brain Injury Association
International Neuropsychological Society
National Academy of Neuropsychology
National Collegiate Athletic Association
National Athletic Trainers Association
Sport Neuropsychology Society

of Neurology has also begun to hold annual concussion-focused conferences each summer. As concussion care and research continues to expand and evolve, there will likely be many more concussion-specific conferences and professional organizations to meet the growing demand. Other professional organizations focused on concussion are listed in Exhibit 8.3. Many of these organizations are typically rooted in one medical (e.g., neurosurgery, neurology), allied health (e.g., athletic training) or psychological (e.g., neuropsychology, sport) discipline. As such, their programming and focus is likely to reflect a bias toward their "home" discipline. However, some organizations such as the American College of Sports Medicine and International Brain Injury Association provide interdisciplinary programming.

CONTINUING THE GROWTH IN CONCUSSION
SPECIALTY CLINICS

The increased recognition and awareness of concussion has been accompanied by an increased demand for specialty care for patients with this injury. In 2000, Freddie Fu, renown orthopaedic surgeon at the University of Pittsburgh, had the foresight to recruit Mark Lovell and his then postdoctoral fellow and one of the coauthors of this book, Michael "Micky" Collins, from Detroit's Henry Ford Hospital to form one of the first concussion-specific clinics in the United States. Fu saw a logical connection between sports medicine and concussions, which often are the result of sport participation. However, such a specialized clinic was unheard of at that time, and initially the viability of the newly formed clinic was in question. We can remember a visit between Anthony Kontos, Mickey Collins, and Mark Lovell in 2001 to Pittsburgh in their new concussion clinic. There were so few patients during that visit that we had time for a 2-hour lunch and an extended drive around the city in the middle of a clinic day. Collins and Lovell were certain that it was just a matter of time before Fu would come in and say, "OK, we tried this concussion thing, but it just isn't working out."

Fast-forward to 2016, and the UPMC Sports Medicine Concussion Program includes more than 20 clinicians, four postdoctoral fellows, and a host of administrative support staff. The clinic averages nearly 20,000 patient visits per year at five clinic sites (including a concussion-only clinic) in the greater Pittsburgh area. Our evidence-based clinic also includes a dedicated research space, the Concussion Research Laboratory, with a staff of five researchers. Although the UPMC Sports Medicine Concussion Program is atypical and much larger than most programs in the United States (and worldwide for that matter), other similar clinics have cropped up in Boston, Houston, Charlotte, Phoenix, and other communities.

Concussions are often first treated by emergency department, primary care, and pediatric physicians, with secondary follow-ups at concussion specific clinics only occurring in larger urban areas with access to these specialized facilities. But as concussion awareness and an understanding of its effects and the importance of early and targeted treatment become commonplace, so too will the availability of concussion specialty clinics. Until then, we advocate for concussion training as a standard part of primary care, pediatric, sports medicine, and emergency medicine training.

CHANGING THE CULTURE OF CONCUSSION

The culture of sports-related concussion, especially at the elite level, needs a renewed direction focused on player health rather than game outcome. For example, in elite soccer matches, players may continue to play after a concussion because of the substitution rule of the Federation Internationale de Football Association (FIFA), which limits teams to three substitutions during a game plus an additional substitute in overtime and no substituted players returning to the field. In short, substitutions are valuable in soccer and therefore are used sparingly. Unfortunately, with limited substitutions in elite soccer, where outcomes equate to millions of dollars in revenue, concussions continue to be downplayed or overlooked by many players, coaches, and sports medicine staff. For positive change regarding awareness, assessment, and treatment in sports, military, and other populations, we must continue to push to change the culture of concussion in these environments.

ADDING CONCUSSION TO YOUR PRACTICE AND EDUCATION

A growing need for concussion specialty clinics with properly trained clinicians to meet the patient demand for the millions of concussions that occur each year is evident. The cornerstone for any concussion care practice is a competent, licensed health care professional with appropriate training and experience providing and coordinating clinical concussion care. A strong referral network is key to a successful concussion clinical practice. Clinicians lacking a strong referral network for concussion treatment will have less success working with patients with concussion. We recommend that practitioners in rural or geographically isolated areas with limited access to referrals and appropriate ancillary care for concussion establish partnering arrangements with clinicians at a reputable, evidence-based clinic. Moving forward, telehealth may further connect clinicians treating concussion to provide the best possible care for patients.

PERSONAL EXPERIENCE WITH CONCUSSION REINFORCES THE PRINCIPLES FROM THIS BOOK

Toward the end of writing this book, Anthony Kontos's wife had a concussion; in this section he tells her story. The resulting experience and outcomes reflect much of the information from this book regarding the role of risk factors, importance of a comprehensive assessment, utility of clinical profiles to inform active and targeted treatments.

My wife was standing on a soccer field waiting for our son when a female high school soccer player missed a shot on goal; the ball hit my wife's head instead. The ball hit her near the left temple and ear and caused her head to rotate rapidly (according to the partially reliable eyewitness accounts of several 14-year-old boys). By the time she walked back to our car she had a headache and dizziness. After the car ride home, vision problems, essentially ocular-migraine-like symptoms, and nausea had been added to her list of symptoms. The concussion was on a Sunday. My wife teaches preschool and went to work on Monday. When I returned from work on Tuesday I found her lying down on the couch. Going to work had exacerbated her symptoms, and she now reported fatigue and was unable to read or look at her phone without provoking symptoms. Driving also exacerbated her ocular and vestibular symptoms. As a result, I did not really need to convince her to come to our clinic the next morning; we both knew that she needed to be evaluated.

It is important to note that my wife has a history of migraine with ocular symptoms, as well as motion sickness. Not surprisingly, her concussion magnified these factors and resulted in a complicated presentation. Fortunately, the results of a thorough clinical interview; medical and injury history; and a comprehensive assessment that included symptoms, computerized neurocognitive, vestibular and oculomotor, and exertion testing identified the relevant risk factors and clinical profiles. Namely, her concussion involved posttraumatic migraine, oculomotor, and vestibular components; as evident by her symptoms and impairment on the visual motion sensitivity and vestibulo-ocular reflex components of the vestibular and oculomotor screening, and design memory, reaction time, and processing speed of the neurocognitive testing. Dynamic exertion, not aerobic exertion, exacerbated her dizziness, nausea, and headache.

Mickey Collins (the second author of this book and her treating clinician) worked together with the multidisciplinary team of vestibular and exertion therapists and sports medicine physicians to develop an active, targeted treatment plan. Initially, my wife was removed from work for two days, because her symptoms were exacerbated from being in a loud, visually stimulating classroom full of rambunctious preschoolers. Following this brief respite, the treatment plan consisted of prescribed low-level physical exertion (i.e., brisk walking on flat ground, always an issue in the hills of Pittsburgh!), as well as vestibular and oculomotor exercises. In addition, because her symptoms were disrupting her sleep, she was prescribed melatonin to help regulate her sleep.

Within a couple of days her symptoms had decreased, and her sleep quality had regulated back to normal. A week later, she was seen for follow-up and her exercises and therapies were accelerated. By her third appointment, approximately 3½ weeks following the injury, she was nearly back to normal on all outcomes, reported low-level symptoms, and had resumed full activities without any return of symptoms. Her recovery is complete, and she has had no recurrent issues associated with her injury. We believe this case, as well as those cases presented in Chapter 6, illustrates many of the principles from this book and reinforces key aspects of good clinical concussion care.

CONCLUSION

We are excited about the direction in which the field of concussion is headed. Advances in awareness, assessment, and treatment, together with an increased understanding of psychological sequelae and at-risk populations, have accelerated the development of the concussion field in recent years. As our understanding of this injury evolves, we believe that the focus of both research and clinical work will move toward active and targeted treatment-based interventions. A growing chorus of clinicians and researchers agree that concussion is treatable and support a paradigm shift toward active and targeted treatments. Funding sources (NIH, CDC, DoD, industry) need to expand support of RCTs to assess the effectiveness of these treatments. Clinical programs should partner with researchers to assess new approaches to treatment in a systematic and evidence-based manner. Otherwise, we risk perpetuating the consensus-driven, rest-based management paradigms that have prevailed over the past decade. As we move toward evidence-based treatments, we need to leverage clinical outcomes research involving metadata to inform our approaches. In the meantime, we should continue fostering awareness of concussion that promotes behavior change to increase reporting and clinical care. The culture surrounding concussion, especially in sports and the military, should support seeking care and reporting concussions.

We hope that the brief cases in this book have provided a summary context for the approach we advocate. We encourage the reader to stay up-to-date on empirical developments and clinical advances in this rapidly evolving field.

REFERENCES

Abaji, J. P., Curnier, D., Moore, R. D., & Ellemberg, D. (2016). Persisting effects of concussion on heart rate variability during physical exertion. *Journal of Neurotrauma, 33*, 811–817. http://dx.doi.org/10.1089/neu.2015.3989

Allen, C., Glasziou, P., & Del Mar, C. (1999). Bed rest: A potentially harmful treatment needing more careful evaluation. *Lancet, 354*(9186), 1229–1233. http://dx.doi.org/10.1016/S0140-6736(98)10063-6

Alsalaheen, B. A., Mucha, A., Morris, L. O., Whitney, S. L., Furman, J. M., Camiolo-Reddy, C. E., . . . Sparto, P. J. (2010). Vestibular rehabilitation for dizziness and balance disorders after concussion. *Journal of Neurologic Physical Therapy, 34*(2), 87–93. http://dx.doi.org/10.1097/NPT.0b013e3181dde568

Alsalaheen, B. A., Stockdale, K., Pechumer, D., & Broglio, S. P. (2016). Measurement error in the Immediate Postconcussion Assessment and Cognitive Testing (ImPACT): Systematic review. *Journal of Head Trauma and Rehabilitation, 31*, 242–251.

Al Sayegh, A., Sandford, D., & Carson, A. J. (2010). Psychological approaches to treatment of postconcussion syndrome: A systematic review. *Journal of Neurology, Neurosurgery, and Psychiatry, 81*, 1128–1134. http://dx.doi.org/10.1136/jnnp.2008.170092

American College of Sports Medicine. (2011). *Concussion in sports.* Retrieved from https://www.acsm.org/docs/brochures/concussion-in-sports.pdf

American Psychological Association. (n.d.). *The concussion toolkit for psychologists.* Retrieved from http://www.ucdenver.edu/academics/colleges/medicalschool/departments/pmr/documents/concussion_toolkit/index.htm

Arfanakis, K., Haughton, V. M., Carew, J. D., Rogers, B. P., Dempsey, R. J., & Meyerand, M. E. (2002). Diffusion tensor MR imaging in diffuse axonal injury. *American Journal of Neuroradiology, 23*, 794–802.

Azulay, J., Smart, C. M., Mott, T., & Cicerone, K. D. (2013). A pilot study examining the effect of mindfulness-based stress reduction on symptoms of chronic mild traumatic brain injury/postconcussive syndrome. *The Journal of Head Trauma Rehabilitation, 28*, 323–331. http://dx.doi.org/10.1097/HTR.0b013e318250ebda

Babcock, L., Yuan, W., Leach, J., Nash, T., & Wade, S. (2015). White matter alterations in youth with acute mild traumatic brain injury. *Journal of Pediatric Rehabilitation Medicine, 8*(4), 285–296. http://dx.doi.org/10.3233/PRM-150347

Babor, T. F., de la Fuente, J. R., Saunders, J., & Grant, M. (1992). *AUDIT: The Alcohol Use Disorders Identification Test: Guidelines for use in primary health care.* Geneva, Switzerland: World Health Organization.

Baker, J. G., Freitas, M. S., Leddy, J. J., Kozlowski, K. F., & Willer, B. S. (2012). Return to full functioning after graded exercise assessment and progressive exercise treatment of postconcussion syndrome. *Rehabilitation Research and Practice, 2012,* Article ID 705309. http://dx.doi.org/10.1155/2012/705309

Barr, W. B., & McCrea, M. (2001). Sensitivity and specificity of standardized neurocognitive testing immediately following sports concussion. *Journal of the International Neuropsychological Society, 7,* 693–702. http://dx.doi.org/10.1017/S1355617701766052

Barth, J. T., Freeman, J. R., Broshek, D. K., & Varney, R. N. (2001). Acceleration-deceleration sport-related concussion: The gravity of it all. *Journal of Athletic Training, 36,* 253–256.

Bazarian, J. J., Blyth, B., & Cimpello, L. (2006). Bench to bedside: Evidence for brain injury after concussion—looking beyond the computed tomography scan. *Academic Emergency Medicine, 13,* 199–214.

Bazarian, J. J., Pope, C., McClung, J., Cheng, Y. T., & Flesher, W. (2003). Ethnic and racial disparities in emergency department care for mild traumatic brain injury. *Academic Emergency Medicine, 10,* 1209–1217. http://dx.doi.org/10.1111/j.1553-2712.2003.tb00605.x

Bazarian, J. J., Zhong, J., Blyth, B., Zhu, T., Kavcic, V., & Peterson, D. (2007). Diffusion tensor imaging detects clinically important axonal damage after mild traumatic brain injury: A pilot study. *Journal of Neurotrauma, 24,* 1447–1459. http://dx.doi.org/10.1089/neu.2007.0241

Beck, A. T., Epstein, N., Brown, G., & Steer, R. A. (1988). An inventory for measuring clinical anxiety: Psychometric properties. *Journal of Consulting and Clinical Psychology, 56,* 893–897.

Beck, A. T., Steer, R. A., & Brown, G. K. (1996). *Manual for the Beck Depression Inventory–II.* San Antonio, TX: Psychological Corporation.

Bedard, A. C., Nichols, S., Barbosa, J. A., Schachar, R., Logan, G. D., & Tannock, R. (2002). The development of selective inhibitory control across the life span. *Developmental Neuropsychology, 21*(1), 93–111. http://dx.doi.org/10.1207/S15326942DN2101_5

Belanger, H. G., Proctor-Weber, Z., Kretzmer, T., Kim, M., French, L. M., & Vanderploeg, R. D. (2011). Symptom complaints following reports of blast versus non-blast mild TBI: Does mechanism of injury matter? *The Clinical Neuropsychologist, 25,* 702–715. http://dx.doi.org/10.1080/13854046.2011.566892

Bey, T., & Ostick, B. (2009). Second impact syndrome. *The Western Journal of Emergency Medicine, 10*(1), 6–10.

Biagas, K. V., Grundl, P. D., Kochanek, P. M., Schiding, J. K., & Nemoto, E. M. (1996). Posttraumatic hyperemia in immature, mature, and aged rats: Autoradiographic determination of cerebral blood flow. *Journal of Neurotrauma, 13*(4), 189–200.

Binder, L. M., Rohling, M. L., & Larrabee, G. J. (1997). A review of mild head trauma. Part I: Meta-analytic review of neuropsychological studies. *Journal of Clinical and Experimental Neuropsychology, 19,* 421–431. http://dx.doi.org/10.1080/01688639708403870

Bloom, G. A., Horton, A. S., McCrory, P., & Johnston, K. M. (2004). Sport psychology and concussion: New impacts to explore. *British Journal of Sports Medicine, 38*, 519–521. http://dx.doi.org/10.1136/bjsm.2004.011999

Boone, K. B., Lu, P., Back, C., King, C., Lee, A., Philpott, L., . . . Warner-Chacon, K. (2002). Sensitivity and specificity of the Rey Dot Counting Test in patients with poor effort and various clinical samples. *Archives of Clinical Neuropsychology, 17*, 625–642.

Brenner, D. J., & Hall, E. J. (2007). Computed tomography—an increasing source of radiation exposure. *The New England Journal of Medicine, 357*, 2277–2284. http://dx.doi.org/10.1056/NEJMra072149

Brody, D. L. (2014). *Concussion care manual.* Oxford, UK: Oxford University Press. http://dx.doi.org/10.1093/med/9780199383863.001.0001

Broglio, S. P., Cantu, R. C., Gioia, G. A., Guskiewicz, K. M., Kutcher, J., Palm, M., . . . the National Athletic Trainers' Association. (2014). National Athletic Trainers' Association position statement: Management of sport concussion. *Journal of Athletic Training, 49*, 245–265. http://dx.doi.org/10.4085/1062-6050-49.1.07

Broglio, S. P., Collins, M. W., Williams, R. M., Mucha, A., & Kontos, A. P. (2015). Current and emerging rehabilitation for concussion: A review of the evidence. *Clinics in Sports Medicine, 34*, 213–231. http://dx.doi.org/10.1016/j.csm.2014.12.005

Broglio, S. P., Eckner, J. T., & Kutcher, J. S. (2012). Field-based measures of head impacts in high school football athletes. *Current Opinion in Pediatrics, 24*, 702–708. http://dx.doi.org/10.1097/MOP.0b013e3283595616

Broglio, S. P., Eckner, J. T., Martini, D., Sosnoff, J. J., Kutcher, J. S., & Randolph, C. (2011). Cumulative head impact burden in high school football. *Journal of Neurotrauma, 28*, 2069–2078. http://dx.doi.org/10.1089/neu.2011.1825

Broglio, S. P., Macciocchi, S. N., & Ferrara, M. S. (2007). Sensitivity of the concussion assessment battery. *Neurosurgery, 60*, 1050–1058. http://dx.doi.org/10.1227/01.NEU.0000255479.90999.C0

Broglio, S. P., Schnebel, B., Sosnoff, J. J., Shin, S., Feng, X., He, X., & Zimmerman, J. (2010). The biomechanical properties of concussions in high school football. *Medicine and Science in Sports and Exercise, 42*, 2064–2071. http://dx.doi.org/10.1249/MSS.0b013e3181dd9156

Broglio, S. P., Sosnoff, J. J., Shin, S., He, X., Alcaraz, C., & Zimmerman, J. (2009). Head impacts during high school football: A biomechanical assessment. *Journal of Athletic Training, 44*, 342–349.

Broglio, S. P., Tomporowski, P. D., & Ferrara, M. S. (2005). Balance performance with a cognitive task: A dual-task testing paradigm. *Medicine and Science in Sports and Exercise, 37*, 689–695. http://dx.doi.org/10.1249/01.MSS.0000159019.14919.09

Broglio, S. P., Williams, R. M., O'Connor, K. L., & Goldstick, J. (2016). Football players' head-impact exposure after limiting of full-contact practices. *Journal of Athletic Training, 51*, 511–518. http://dx.doi.org/10.4085/1062-6050-51.7.04

Broshek, D. K., Kaushik, T., Freeman, J. R., Erlanger, D., Webbe, F., & Barth, J. T. (2005). Sex differences in outcome following sports-related concussion. *Journal of Neurosurgery, 102,* 856–863. http://dx.doi.org/10.3171/jns.2005.102.5.0856

Brown, N. J., Mannix, R. C., O'Brien, M. J., Gostine, D., Collins, M. W., & Meehan, W. P., III. (2014). Effect of cognitive activity level on duration of post-concussion symptoms. *Pediatrics, 133*(2), e299–e304. http://dx.doi.org/10.1542/peds.2013-2125

Browning, M., Shear, D. A., Bramlett, H. M., Dixon, C. E., Mondello, S., Schmid, K. E., . . . Kochanek, P. M. (2016). Levetiracetam treatment in traumatic brain injury: Operation brain trauma therapy. *Journal of Neurotrauma, 33,* 581–594. http://dx.doi.org/10.1089/neu.2015.4131

Bryan, M. A., Rowhani-Rahbar, A., Comstock, R. D., Rivara, F., & the Seattle Sports Concussion Research Collaborative. (2016). Sports- and recreation-related concussions in US youth. *Pediatrics, 138*(1), e20154635. http://dx.doi.org/10.1542/peds.2015-4635

Byrnes, K. R., Wilson, C. M., Brabazon, F., von Leden, R., Jurgens, J. S., Oakes, T. R., & Selwyn, R. G. (2014). FDG-PET imaging in mild traumatic brain injury: A critical review. *Frontiers in Neuroenergetics, 5,* 13. http://dx.doi.org/10.3389/fnene.2013.00013

Cacioppo, J. T., Hawkley, L. C., Norman, G. J., & Berntson, G. G. (2011). Social isolation. *Annals of the New York Academy of Sciences, 1231,* 17–22. http://dx.doi.org/10.1111/j.1749-6632.2011.06028.x

Cantu, R. C. (1986). Guidelines for return to contact sports after a cerebral concussion. *The Physician and Sportsmedicine, 14*(10), 75–83. http://dx.doi.org/10.1080/00913847.1986.11709197

Cantu, R. C. (1992). Cerebral concussion in sport. Management and prevention. *Sports Medicine, 14*(1), 64–74. http://dx.doi.org/10.2165/00007256-199214010-00005

Cantu, R. C. (1998). Second-impact syndrome. *Clinics in Sports Medicine, 17*(1), 37–44. http://dx.doi.org/10.1016/S0278-5919(05)70059-4

Cantu, R. C. (2001). Posttraumatic retrograde and anterograde amnesia: Pathophysiology and implications in grading and safe return to play. *Journal of Athletic Training, 36,* 244–248.

Cantu, R. C., & Gean, A. D. (2010). Second-impact syndrome and a small subdural hematoma: An uncommon catastrophic result of repetitive head injury with a characteristic imaging appearance. *Journal of Neurotrauma, 27,* 1557–1564. http://dx.doi.org/10.1089/neu.2010.1334

Cantu, R. C., & Voy, R. (1995). Second impact syndrome a risk in any contact sport. *Physicians and Sportsmedicine, 23,* 27–34.

Cao, C., Tutwiler, R. L., & Slobounov, S. (2008). Automatic classification of athletes with residual functional deficits following concussion by means of EEG signal using support vector machine. *IEEE Transactions on Neural Systems and Rehabilitation Engineering, 16,* 327–335. http://dx.doi.org/10.1109/TNSRE.2008.918422

Carr, W., Polejaeva, E., Grome, A., Crandall, B., LaValle, C., Eonta, S. E., & Young, L. A. (2015). Relation of repeated low-level blast exposure with symptomology similar to concussion. *The Journal of Head Trauma Rehabilitation, 30*(1), 47–55. http://dx.doi.org/10.1097/HTR.0000000000000064

Carter, T., Morres, I. D., Meade, O., & Callaghan, P. (2016). The effect of exercise on depressive symptoms in adolescents: A systematic review and meta-analysis. *Journal of the American Academy of Child & Adolescent Psychiatry, 55,* 580–590. http://dx.doi.org/10.1016/j.jaac.2016.04.016

Cassidy, J. D., Cancelliere, C., Carroll, L. J., Côté, P., Hincapié, C. A., Holm, L. W., . . . Borg, J. (2014). Systematic review of self-reported prognosis in adults after mild traumatic brain injury: Results of the International Collaboration on Mild Traumatic Brain Injury Prognosis. *Archives of Physical Medicine and Rehabilitation, 95*(3, Suppl.), S132–S151. http://dx.doi.org/10.1016/j.apmr.2013.08.299

Casson, I. R., Sethi, N. K., & Meehan, W. P., III. (2015). Early symptom burden predicts recovery after sport-related concussion. *Neurology, 85*(1), 110–111. http://dx.doi.org/10.1212/WNL.0000000000001700

Centers for Disease Control and Prevention. (2017). *Heads up.* Retrieved from https://www.cdc.gov/headsup/index.html

Chafetz, M. (2011). The psychological consultative examination for Social Security disability. *Psychological Injury and Law, 4,* 235–244. http://dx.doi.org/10.1007/s12207-011-9112-5

Chen, J. K., Johnston, K. M., Petrides, M., & Ptito, A. (2008). Neural substrates of symptoms of depression following concussion in male athletes with persisting postconcussion symptoms. *Archives of General Psychiatry, 65*(1), 81–89. http://dx.doi.org/10.1001/archgenpsychiatry.2007.8

Choe, M. C., & Giza, C. C. (2015). Diagnosis and management of acute concussion. *Seminar in Neurology, 35,* 29–41.

Chrisman, S. P., Rivara, F. P., Schiff, M. A., Zhou, C., & Comstock, R. D. (2013). Risk factors for concussive symptoms 1 week or longer in high school athletes. *Brain Injury, 27*(1), 1–9. http://dx.doi.org/10.3109/02699052.2012.722251

Clarke, L. A., Genat, R. C., & Anderson, J. F. I. (2012). Long-term cognitive complaint and post-concussive symptoms following mild traumatic brain injury: The role of cognitive and affective factors. *Brain Injury, 26,* 298–307. http://dx.doi.org/10.3109/02699052.2012.654588

Clement, D., & Shannon, V. R. (2011). Injured athletes' perceptions about social support. *Journal of Sport Rehabilitation, 20,* 457–470. http://dx.doi.org/10.1123/jsr.20.4.457

Collie, A., Maruff, P., Darby, D. G., & McStephen, M. (2003). The effects of practice on the cognitive test performance of neurologically normal individuals assessed at brief test–retest intervals. *Journal of the International Neuropsychological Society, 9*, 419–428.

Collins, C. L., Fletcher, E. N., Fields, S. K., Kluchurosky, L., Rohrkemper, M. K., Comstock, R. D., & Cantu, R. C. (2014). Neck strength: A protective factor reducing risk for concussion in high school sports. *The Journal of Primary Prevention, 35*, 309–319. http://dx.doi.org/10.1007/s10935-014-0355-2

Collins, M. W. (2015). *How knowledgeable are Americans about concussions? Assessing and recalibrating the public's knowledge.* Retrieved from http://rethinkconcussions.upmc.com/wp-content/uploads/2015/09/harris-poll-report.pdf

Collins, M. W., Grindel, S. H., Lovell, M. R., Dede, D. E., Moser, D. J., Phalin, B. R., . . . McKeag, D. B. (1999). Relationship between concussion and neuropsychological performance in college football players. *Journal of the American Medical Association, 282*, 964–970. http://dx.doi.org/10.1001/jama.282.10.964

Collins, M. W., Iverson, G. L., Lovell, M. R., McKeag, D. B., Norwig, J., & Maroon, J. (2003). On-field predictors of neuropsychological and symptom deficit following sports-related concussion. *Clinical Journal of Sport Medicine, 13*(4), 222–229. http://dx.doi.org/10.1097/00042752-200307000-00005

Collins, M. W., Kontos, A. P., Okonkwo, D. O., Almquist, J., Bailes, J., Barisa, M., . . . Zafonte, R. (2016). Statements of agreement from the Targeted Evaluation and Active Management (TEAM) approaches to treating concussion meeting held in Pittsburgh, October 15–16, 2015. *Neurosurgery, 79*, 912–929. http://dx.doi.org/10.1227/NEU.0000000000001447

Collins, M. W., Kontos, A. P., Reynolds, E., Murawski, C. D., & Fu, F. H. (2014). A comprehensive, targeted approach to the clinical care of athletes following sport-related concussion. *Knee Surgery, Sports Traumatology, Arthroscopy, 22*, 235–246. http://dx.doi.org/10.1007/s00167-013-2791-6

Collins, M. W., Lovell, M. R., & McKeag, D. B. (1999). Current issues in managing sports-related concussion. *Journal of the American Medical Association, 282*, 2283–2285. http://dx.doi.org/10.1001/jama.282.24.2283

Colloca, L., & Finniss, D. (2012). Nocebo effects, patient-clinician communication, and therapeutic outcomes. *Journal of the American Medical Association, 307*, 567–568. http://dx.doi.org/10.1001/jama.2012.115

Colvin, A. C., Mullen, J., Lovell, M. R., West, R. V., Collins, M. W., & Groh, M. (2009). The role of concussion history and gender in recovery from soccer-related concussion. *The American Journal of Sports Medicine, 37*, 1699–1704. http://dx.doi.org/10.1177/0363546509332497

Concussion Vital Signs. (n.d.). *Concussion vital signs resource portal* [Website]. Retrieved from http://www.concussionvitalsigns.com/Resources.html

Conder, R., & Conder, A. A. (2015). Neuropsychological and psychological rehabilitation interventions in refractory sport-related post-concussive syndrome. *Brain Injury, 29*, 249–262. http://dx.doi.org/10.3109/02699052.2014.965209

Cornish, P. J., Blanchard, E. B., & Jaccard, J. (1995). Test–retest reliability of 24-hour ambulatory blood pressures. *Biofeedback and Self-Regulation, 20*(2), 137–154. http://dx.doi.org/10.1007/BF01720970

Corrigan, J. D., & Bogner, J. (2007). Initial reliability and validity of the Ohio State University TBI Identification Method. *The Journal of Head Trauma Rehabilitation, 22,* 318–329. http://dx.doi.org/10.1097/01.HTR.0000300227.67748.77

Covassin, T., Crutcher, B., Bleecker, A., Heiden, E. O., Dailey, A., & Yang, J. (2014). Postinjury anxiety and social support among collegiate athletes: A comparison between orthopaedic injuries and concussions. *Journal of Athletic Training, 49,* 462–468. http://dx.doi.org/10.4085/1062-6059-49.2.03

Covassin, T., & Elbin, R. J. (2011). The female athlete: The role of gender in the assessment and management of sport-related concussion. *Clinics in Sports Medicine, 30*(1), 125–131. http://dx.doi.org/10.1016/j.csm.2010.08.001

Covassin, T., Elbin, R. J., Bleecker, A., Lipchik, A., & Kontos, A. P. (2013). Are there differences in neurocognitive function and symptoms between male and female soccer players after concussions? *The American Journal of Sports Medicine, 41,* 2890–2895. http://dx.doi.org/10.1177/0363546513509962

Covassin, T., Elbin, R. J., Crutcher, B., & Burkhart, S. (2013). The management of sport-related concussion: Considerations for male and female athletes. *Translational Stroke Research, 4,* 420–424. http://dx.doi.org/10.1007/s12975-012-0228-z

Covassin, T., Elbin, R. J., Harris, W., Parker, T., & Kontos, A. (2012). The role of age and sex in symptoms, neurocognitive performance, and postural stability in athletes after concussion. *The American Journal of Sports Medicine, 40,* 1303–1312. http://dx.doi.org/10.1177/0363546512444554

Covassin, T., Elbin, R. J., Larson, E., & Kontos, A. P. (2012). Sex and age differences in depression and baseline sport-related concussion neurocognitive performance and symptoms. *Clinical Journal of Sport Medicine, 22*(2), 98–104. http://dx.doi.org/10.1097/JSM.0b013e31823403d2

Covassin, T., Stearne, D., & Elbin, R. J. (2008). Concussion history and postconcussion neurocognitive performance and symptoms in collegiate athletes. *Journal of Athletic Training, 43,* 119–124. http://dx.doi.org/10.4085/1062-6050-43.2.119

Covassin, T., Weiss, L., Powell, J., Womack, C., & Lovell, M. R. (2007). Effects of a maximal exercise test on neurocognitive function. *British Journal of Sports Medicine, 41,* 370–374. http://dx.doi.org/10.1136/bjsm.2006.032334

Craton, N., & Leslie, O. (2014). Is rest the best intervention for concussion? Lessons learned from the whiplash model. *Current Sports Medicine Reports, 13*(4), 201–204. http://dx.doi.org/10.1249/JSR.0000000000000072

Cubon, V. A., Putukian, M., Boyer, C., & Dettwiler, A. (2011). A diffusion tensor imaging study on the white matter skeleton in individuals with sports-related concussion. *Journal of Neurotrauma, 28*(2), 189–201. http://dx.doi.org/10.1089/neu.2010.1430

Currie, D. W., Comstock, R. D., Fields, S. K., & Cantu, R. C. (2017). A paired comparison of initial and recurrent concussions sustained by US high school athletes within a single athletic season. *The Journal of Head Trauma Rehabilitation*, *32*, 90–97.

Custer, A., Sufrinko, A., Elbin, R. J., Covassin, T., Collins, M. W., & Kontos, A. P. (2016). High baseline postconcussion symptom scores and outcomes in athletes. *Journal of Athletic Training*, *51*, 136–141. http://dx.doi.org/10.4085/1062-6050-51.2.12

Czerniak, S. M., Sikoglu, E. M., Liso Navarro, A. A., McCafferty, J., Eisenstock, J., Stevenson, J. H., . . . Moore, C. M. (2015). A resting state functional magnetic resonance imaging study of concussion in collegiate athletes. *Brain Imaging and Behavior*, *9*, 323–332. http://dx.doi.org/10.1007/s11682-014-9312-1

Dash, P. K., Zhao, J., Hergenroeder, G., & Moore, A. N. (2010). Biomarkers for the diagnosis, prognosis, and evaluation of treatment efficacy for traumatic brain injury. *Neurotherapeutics; The Journal of the American Society for Experimental NeuroTherapeutics*, *7*(1), 100–114. http://dx.doi.org/10.1016/j.nurt.2009.10.019

Davis, G. A., Anderson, V., Babl, F. E., Gioia, G., Giza, C. G., Meehan, W., . . . Zemek, R. (2017). What is the difference in concussion management in children as compared with adults? A systematic review. *British Journal of Sports Medicine*, *51*, 949–957.

Davis, G. A., Castellani, R. J., & McCrory, P. (2015). Neurodegeneration and sport. *Neurosurgery*, *76*, 643–655; discussion 655-646. http://dx.doi.org/10.1227/NEU.0000000000000722

Davis, G. A., Iverson, G. L., Guskiewicz, K. M., Ptito, A., & Johnston, K. M. (2009). Contributions of neuroimaging, balance testing, electrophysiology and blood markers to the assessment of sport-related concussion. *British Journal of Sports Medicine*, *43*(Suppl. 1), i36–i45. http://dx.doi.org/10.1136/bjsm.2009.058123

de Courten-Myers, G. M. (1999). The human cerebral cortex: Gender differences in structure and function. *Journal of Neuropathology & Experimental Neurology*, *58*, 217–226.

de Kruijk, J. R., Leffers, P., Meerhoff, S., Rutten, J., & Twijnstra, A. (2002). Effectiveness of bed rest after mild traumatic brain injury: A randomised trial of no versus six days of bed rest. *Journal of Neurology, Neurosurgery & Psychiatry*, *73*, 167–172. http://dx.doi.org/10.1136/jnnp.73.2.167

Defense and Veterans Brain Injury Center. (2012). *Military acute concussion evaluation*. Retrieved from https://www.jsomonline.org/TBI/MACE_Revised_2012.pdf

Defense and Veterans Brain Injury Center. (2017). *DoD worldwide numbers for TBI*. Retrieved from https://dvbic.dcoe.mil/dod-worldwide-numbers-tbi

de Lanerolle, N. C., Hamid, H., Kulas, J., Pan, J. W., Czlapinski, R., Rinaldi, A., . . . Hetherington, H. P. (2014). Concussive brain injury from explosive blast. *Annals of Clinical and Translational Neurology*, *1*, 692–702.

Dematteo, C., Volterman, K. A., Breithaupt, P. G., Claridge, E. A., Adamich, J., & Timmons, B. W. (2015). Exertion testing in youth with mild traumatic brain injury/concussion. *Medicine and Science in Sports and Exercise, 47*, 2283–2290. http://dx.doi.org/10.1249/MSS.0000000000000682

Derogatis, L. R. (1993). *BSI Brief Symptom Inventory: Administration, scoring, and procedure manual* (4th ed.). Minneapolis, MN: National Computer Systems.

Derogatis, L. R. (2001). *Brief Symptom Inventory 18 (BSI-18): Administration, scoring, and procedures manual*. Bloomington, MN: Pearson.

DiFeo, G., & Shors, T. J. (2017). Mental and physical skill training increases neurogenesis via cell survival in the adolescent hippocampus. *Brain Research, 1654*(Pt B), 95–101. http://dx.doi.org/10.1016/j.brainres.2016.08.015

Dorminy, M., Hoogeveen, A., Tierney, R. T., Higgins, M., McDevitt, J. K., & Kretzschmar, J. (2015). Effect of soccer heading ball speed on S100B, sideline concussion assessments and head impact kinematics. *Brain Injury, 25*, 1–7.

Eagan Brown, B., & Vaccaro, M. (2014). Pennsylvania's BrainSTEPS program: The return to school and academics statewide concussion management team (CMT) project. *Brain Injury, 28*, 838–839.

Echemendia, R. J., Meeuwisse, W., McCrory, P., Davis, G. A., Putukian, M., Leddy, J., . . . Herring, S. (2017). The Sport Concussion Assessment Tool 5th Edition (SCAT5): Background and rationale. *British Journal of Sports Medicine, 51*, 848–850.

Eckner, J. T., Rettmann, A., Narisetty, N., Greer, J., Moore, B., Brimacombe, S., . . . Broglio, S. P. (2016). Stability of an ERP-based measure of brain network activation (BNA) in athletes: A new electrophysiological assessment tool for concussion. *Brain Injury, 30*, 1075–1081. http://dx.doi.org/10.3109/02699052.2016.1160152

Eckner, J. T., Sabin, M., Kutcher, J. S., & Broglio, S. P. (2011). No evidence for a cumulative impact effect on concussion injury threshold. *Journal of Neurotrauma, 28*, 2079–2090. http://dx.doi.org/10.1089/neu.2011.1910

Eierud, C., Craddock, R. C., Fletcher, S., Aulakh, M., King-Casas, B., Kuehl, D., & LaConte, S. M. (2014). Neuroimaging after mild traumatic brain injury: Review and meta-analysis. *NeuroImage: Clinical, 4*, 283–294. http://dx.doi.org/10.1016/j.nicl.2013.12.009

Elbin, R. J., Beatty, A., Covassin, T., Schatz, P., Hydeman, A., & Kontos, A. P. (2015). A preliminary examination of neurocognitive performance and symptoms following a bout of soccer heading in athletes wearing protective soccer headbands. *Research in Sports Medicine, 23*(2), 203–214. http://dx.doi.org/10.1080/15438627.2015.1005293

Elbin, R. J., Covassin, T., Hakun, J., Kontos, A. P., Berger, K., Pfeiffer, K., & Ravizza, S. (2012). Do brain activation changes persist in athletes with a history of multiple concussions who are asymptomatic? *Brain Injury, 26*, 1217–1225. http://dx.doi.org/10.3109/02699052.2012.672788

Elbin, R. J., Knox, J., Kegel, N., Schatz, A. P., Lowder, H., French, J., . . . Kontos, A. P. (2016). Assessing symptoms in adolescents following sport-related concussion: A comparison of four different approaches. *Applied Neuropsychology: Child, 5,* 294–302. http://dx.doi.org/10.1080/21622965.2015.1077334

Elbin, R. J., Sufrinko, A., Schatz, P., French, J., Collins, M. W., & Kontos, A. P. (2016). Athletes that continue to play with sport-related concussion demonstrate prolonged recovery and worse outcomes: 1907 Board #59 June 2, 2:00 PM–3:30 PM. *Medicine and Science in Sports and Exercise, 48*(5, Suppl. 1), 525. http://dx.doi.org/10.1249/01.mss.0000486580.32473.21

Elbin, R. J., Sufrinko, A., Schatz, P., French, J., Henry, L., Burkhart, S., . . . Kontos, A. P. (2016). Removal from play after concussion and recovery time. *Pediatrics, 138*(3), e20160910.

Ellis, M. J., Leddy, J. J., & Willer, B. (2015). Physiological, vestibulo-ocular and cervicogenic post-concussion disorders: An evidence-based classification system with directions for treatment. *Brain Injury, 29,* 238–248.

Ellis, M. J., Ritchie, L. J., Koltek, M., Hosain, S., Cordingley, D., Chu, S., . . . Russell, K. (2015). Psychiatric outcomes after pediatric sports-related concussion. *Journal of Neurosurgery. Pediatrics, 16,* 709–718. http://dx.doi.org/10.3171/2015.5.PEDS15220

Emerson, C. S., Headrick, J. P., & Vink, R. (1993). Estrogen improves biochemical and neurologic outcome following traumatic brain injury in male rats, but not in females. *Brain Research, 608*(1), 95–100. http://dx.doi.org/10.1016/0006-8993(93)90778-L

Erdal, K. (2012). Neuropsychological testing for sports-related concussion: How athletes can sandbag their baseline testing without detection. *Archives of Clinical Neuropsychology, 27,* 473–479. http://dx.doi.org/10.1093/arclin/acs050

Erlanger, D., Feldman, D., Kutner, K., Kaushik, T., Kroger, H., Festa, J., Barth, J., Freeman, J., & Broshek, D. (2003). Development and validation of a web-based neuropsychological test protocol for sports-related return-to-play decision-making. *Archives of Clinical Neuropsychology, 18*(3), 293–316.

Erlanger, D., Kaushik, T., Cantu, R., Barth, J. T., Broshek, D. K., Freeman, J. R., & Webbe, F. M. (2003). Symptom-based assessment of the severity of a concussion. *Journal of Neurosurgery, 98,* 477–484. http://dx.doi.org/10.3171/jns.2003.98.3.0477

Esposito, G., Van Horn, J. D., Weinberger, D. R., & Berman, K. F. (1996). Gender differences in cerebral blood flow as a function of cognitive state with PET. *Journal of Nuclear Medicine, 37,* 559–564.

Evans, L., Hardy, L., & Fleming, S. (2000). Intervention strategies with injured athletes: An action research study. *The Sport Psychologist, 14,* 188–206. http://dx.doi.org/10.1123/tsp.14.2.188

Falleti, M. G., Maruff, P., Collie, A., & Darby, D. G. (2006). Practice effects associated with the repeated assessment of cognitive function using the CogState battery at 10-minute, one week and one month test–retest intervals. *Journal of Clinical and Experimental Neuropsychology, 28,* 1095–1112.

Fazio, V. C., Lovell, M. R., Pardini, J. E., & Collins, M. W. (2007). The relation between postconcussion symptoms and neurocognitive performance in concussed athletes. *NeuroRehabilitation*, *22*(3), 207–216.

Feinstein, A., Ouchterlony, D., Somerville, J., & Jardine, A. (2001). The effects of litigation on symptom expression: A prospective study following mild traumatic brain injury. *Medicine, Science, and the Law*, *41*(2), 116–121. http://dx.doi.org/10.1177/002580240104100206

Field, M., Collins, M. W., Lovell, M. R., & Maroon, J. (2003). Does age play a role in recovery from sports-related concussion? A comparison of high school and collegiate athletes. *The Journal of Pediatrics*, *142*, 546–553. http://dx.doi.org/10.1067/mpd.2003.190

Fingerman, K. L., Cheng, Y. P., Wesselmann, E. D., Zarit, S., Furstenberg, F., & Birditt, K. S. (2012). Helicopter parents and landing pad kids: Intense parental support of grown children. *Journal of Marriage and the Family*, *74*, 880–896. http://dx.doi.org/10.1111/j.1741-3737.2012.00987.x

Finkbeiner, N. W., Max, J. E., Longman, S., & Debert, C. (2016). Knowing what we don't know: Long-term psychiatric outcomes following adult concussion in sports. *The Canadian Journal of Psychiatry*, *61*(5), 270–276. http://dx.doi.org/10.1177/0706743716644953

Fino, P. C., Nussbaum, M. A., & Brolinson, P. G. (2016). Locomotor deficits in recently concussed athletes and matched controls during single and dual-task turning gait: Preliminary results. *Journal of Neuroengineering and Rehabilitation*, *13*(1), 65. http://dx.doi.org/10.1186/s12984-016-0177-y

Folkman, S., & Lazarus, R. S. (1985). If it changes it must be a process: Study of emotion and coping during three stages of a college examination. *Journal of Personality and Social Psychology*, *48*(1), 150–170. http://dx.doi.org/10.1037/0022-3514.48.1.150

Foutch, B. K. (2015). An atypical presentation of visual conversion disorder. *Journal of Optometry*, *8*, 273–275. http://dx.doi.org/10.1016/j.optom.2015.01.006

Fox, Z. G., Mihalik, J. P., Blackburn, J. T., Battaglini, C. L., & Guskiewicz, K. M. (2008). Return of postural control to baseline after anaerobic and aerobic exercise protocols. *Journal of Athletic Training*, *43*, 456–463. http://dx.doi.org/10.4085/1062-6050-43.5.456

Fralick, M., Thiruchelvam, D., Tien, H. C., & Redelmeier, D. A. (2016). Risk of suicide after a concussion. *Canadian Medical Association Journal*, *188*, 497–504. http://dx.doi.org/10.1503/cmaj.150790

Frommer, L. J., Gurka, K. K., Cross, K. M., Ingersoll, C. D., Comstock, R. D., & Saliba, S. A. (2011). Sex differences in concussion symptoms of high school athletes. *Journal of Athletic Training*, *46*, 76–84. http://dx.doi.org/10.4085/1062-6050-46.1.76

Furman, J. M., Raz, Y., & Whitney, S. L. (2010). Geriatric vestibulopathy assessment and management. *Current Opinion in Otolaryngology & Head & Neck Surgery*, *18*, 386–391. http://dx.doi.org/10.1097/MOO.0b013e32833ce5a6

Galetta, K. M., Brandes, L. E., Maki, K., Dziemianowicz, M. S., Laudano, E., Allen, M., . . . Balcer, L. J. (2011). The King-Devick test and sports-related concussion: Study of a rapid visual screening tool in a collegiate cohort. *Journal of the Neurological Sciences, 309*, 34–39. http://dx.doi.org/10.1016/j.jns.2011.07.039

Gavett, B. E., Stern, R. A., & McKee, A. C. (2011). Chronic traumatic encephalopathy: A potential late effect of sport-related concussive and subconcussive head trauma. *Clinics in Sports Medicine, 30*(1), 179–188. http://dx.doi.org/10.1016/j.csm.2010.09.007

Gay, M., Ray, W., Johnson, B., Teel, E., Geronimo, A., & Slobounov, S. (2015). Feasibility of EEG measures in conjunction with light exercise for return-to-play evaluation after sports-related concussion. *Developmental Neuropsychology, 40*, 248–253. http://dx.doi.org/10.1080/87565641.2015.1014486

Gessel, L. M., Fields, S. K., Collins, C. L., Dick, R. W., & Comstock, R. D. (2007). Concussions among United States high school and collegiate athletes. *Journal of Athletic Training, 42*, 495–503.

Giedd, J. N. (2004). Structural magnetic resonance imaging of the adolescent brain. *Annals of the New York Academy of Sciences, 1021*, 77–85. http://dx.doi.org/10.1196/annals.1308.009

Gioia, G. A. (2015). Multimodal evaluation and management of children with concussion: Using our heads and available evidence. *Brain Injury, 29*(2), 195–206. http://dx.doi.org/10.3109/02699052.2014.965210

Gioia, G. A., & Collins, M. W. (2006). Acute Concussion Evaluation (ACE) care plan. *Heads-up: Brain injury in your practice. Centers for Disease Control and Prevention.* Retrieved from https://www.cdc.gov/headsup/pdfs/providers/ace_care_plan_returning_to_work-a.pdf

Gioia, G. A., Glang, A. E., Hooper, S. R., & Brown, B. E. (2016). Building statewide infrastructure for the academic support of students with mild traumatic brain injury. *The Journal of Head Trauma Rehabilitation, 31*, 397–406.

Gioia, G. A., Schneider, J. C., Vaughan, C. G., & Isquith, P. K. (2009). Which symptom assessments and approaches are uniquely appropriate for paediatric concussion? *British Journal of Sports Medicine, 43*(Suppl. 1), i13–i22.

Giza, C. C., Griesbach, G. S., & Hovda, D. A. (2005). Experience-dependent behavioral plasticity is disturbed following traumatic injury to the immature brain. *Behavioural Brain Research, 157*(1), 11–22. http://dx.doi.org/10.1016/j.bbr.2004.06.003

Giza, C. C., & Hovda, D. A. (2001). The neurometabolic cascade of concussion. *Journal of Athletic Training, 36*(3), 228–235.

Giza, C. C., & Hovda, D. A. (2014). The new neurometabolic cascade of concussion. *Neurosurgery, 75*(Suppl. 4), S24–S33. http://dx.doi.org/10.1227/NEU.0000000000000505

Giza, C. C., Kutcher, J. S., Ashwal, S., Barth, J., Getchius, T. S., Gioia, G. A., . . . Zafonte, R. (2013). Summary of evidence-based guideline update: Evaluation and management of concussion in sports: Report of the Guideline Development Subcommittee of the American Academy of Neurology. *Neurology, 80,* 2250–2257. http://dx.doi.org/10.1212/WNL.0b013e31828d57dd

Glang, A. E., Koester, M. C., Chesnutt, J. C., Gioia, G. A., McAvoy, K., Marshall, S., & Gau, J. M. (2015). The effectiveness of a web-based resource in improving postconcussion management in high schools. *The Journal of Adolescent Health, 56*(1), 91–97. http://dx.doi.org/10.1016/j.jadohealth.2014.08.011

Gogtay, N., Giedd, J. N., Lusk, L., Hayashi, K. M., Greenstein, D., Vaituzis, A. C., . . . Thompson, P. M. (2004). Dynamic mapping of human cortical development during childhood through early adulthood. *Proceedings of the National Academy of Sciences of the United States of America, 101,* 8174–8179. http://dx.doi.org/10.1073/pnas.0402680101

Goodglass, H., Kaplan, E., & Weintraub, S. (2001). *Boston Naming Test* (2nd ed., p. 61). Baltimore, MD: Lippincott Williams & Wilkins.

Gordon, K. E., Dooley, J. M., & Wood, E. P. (2006). Is migraine a risk factor for the development of concussion? *British Journal of Sports Medicine, 40*(2), 184–185. http://dx.doi.org/10.1136/bjsm.2005.022251

Govindaraju, V., Gauger, G. E., Manley, G. T., Ebel, A., Meeker, M., & Maudsley, A. A. (2004). Volumetric proton spectroscopic imaging of mild traumatic brain injury. *American Journal of Neuroradiology, 25,* 730–737.

Green, P. (2004). *Green's Medical Symptom Validity Test (MSVT) for Microsoft windows user's manual.* Edmonton, Canada: Green's Publishing.

Griesbach, G. S., Hovda, D. A., Molteni, R., Wu, A., & Gomez-Pinilla, F. (2004). Voluntary exercise following traumatic brain injury: Brain-derived neurotrophic factor upregulation and recovery of function. *Neuroscience, 125*(1), 129–139. http://dx.doi.org/10.1016/j.neuroscience.2004.01.030

Grønli, J., Bramham, C., Murison, R., Kanhema, T., Fiske, E., Bjorvatn, B., . . . Portas, C. M. (2006). Chronic mild stress inhibits BDNF protein expression and CREB activation in the dentate gyrus but not in the hippocampus proper. *Pharmacology, Biochemistry, and Behavior, 85,* 842–849. http://dx.doi.org/10.1016/j.pbb.2006.11.021

Grubenhoff, J. A., Currie, D., Comstock, R. D., Juarez-Colunga, E., Bajaj, L., & Kirkwood, M. W. (2016). Psychological factors associated with delayed symptom resolution in children with concussion. *Journal of Pediatrics, 174,* 27–32. http://dx.doi.org/10.1016/j.jpeds.2016.03.027

Guskiewicz, K. M. (2001). Postural stability assessment following concussion: One piece of the puzzle. *Clinical Journal of Sport Medicine, 11*(3), 182–189. http://dx.doi.org/10.1097/00042752-200107000-00009

Guskiewicz, K. M., Mihalik, J. P., Shankar, V., Marshall, S. W., Crowell, D. H., Oliaro, S. M., . . . Hooker, D. N. (2007). Measurement of head impacts in collegiate football players: Relationship between head impact biomechanics and acute clinical outcome after concussion. *Neurosurgery, 61,* 1244–1252. http://dx.doi.org/10.1227/01.neu.0000306103.68635.1a

Guskiewicz, K. M., Bruce, S. L., Cantu, R. C., Ferrara, M. S., Kelly, J. P., McCrea, M., . . . Valovich McLeod, T. C. (2004). National Athletic Trainers' Association position statement: Management of sport-related concussion. *Journal of Athletic Training, 39*(3), 280–297.

Guskiewicz, K. M., Weaver, N. L., Padua, D. A., & Garrett, W. E., Jr. (2000). Epidemiology of concussion in collegiate and high school football players. *The American Journal of Sports Medicine, 28,* 643–650. http://dx.doi.org/10.1177/03635465000280050401

Haider, A. H., Efron, D. T., Haut, E. R., DiRusso, S. M., Sullivan, T., & Cornwell, E. E., III. (2007). Black children experience worse clinical and functional outcomes after traumatic brain injury: An analysis of the National Pediatric Trauma Registry. *Journal of Trauma-Injury Infection & Critical Care, 62,* 1259–1263. http://dx.doi.org/10.1097/TA.0b013e31803c760e

Hallett, M., Fahn, S., Jankovic, J., Lang, A., Cloninger, C., & Yudofsky, S. (2006). *Psychogenic movement disorders: Neurology and neuropsychiatry.* Philadelphia, PA: Lippincott Williams & Wilkins.

Halstead, M. E., Walter, K. D., & the Council on Sports Medicine and Fitness. (2010). Sport-related concussion in children and adolescents. *Pediatrics, 126,* 597–615. http://dx.doi.org/10.1542/peds.2010-2005

Haran, F. J., Tierney, R., Wright, W. G., Keshner, E., & Silter, M. (2013). Acute changes in postural control after soccer heading. *International Journal of Sports Medicine, 34,* 350–354.

Harmon, K. G., Drezner, J. A., Gammons, M., Guskiewicz, K. M., Halstead, M., Herring, S. A., . . . Roberts, W. O. (2013). American Medical Society for Sports Medicine position statement: Concussion in sport. *British Journal of Sports Medicine, 47,* 15–26.

Harris Poll. (2015). *How knowledgeable are Americans about concussions? Assessing and recalibrating the public's knowledge.* Retrieved from http://rethinkconcussions.upmc.com/wp-content/uploads/2015/09/harris-poll-report.pdf

Hazrati, L.-N., Tartaglia, M. C., Diamandis, P., Davis, K. D., Green, R. E., Wennberg, R., . . . Tator, C. H. (2013). Absence of chronic traumatic encephalopathy in retired football players with multiple concussions and neurological symptomatology. *Frontiers in Human Neuroscience, 7,* 222.

Heath, I. (2013). Overdiagnosis: When good intentions meet vested interests—an essay by Iona Heath. *BMJ, 347,* f6361. http://dx.doi.org/10.1136/bmj.f6361

Henry, L. C., Burkhart, S. O., Elbin, R. J., Agarwal, V., & Kontos, A. P. (2015). Traumatic axonal injury and persistent emotional lability in an adolescent following moderate traumatic brain injury: A case study. *Journal of Clinical and Experimental Neuropsychology, 37,* 439–454. http://dx.doi.org/10.1080/13803395.2015.1025708

Henry, L. C., Elbin, R. J., Collins, M. W., Marchetti, G., & Kontos, A. P. (2016). Examining recovery trajectories after sport-related concussion with a multimodal clinical assessment approach. *Neurosurgery, 78,* 232–241. http://dx.doi.org/10.1227/NEU.0000000000001041

Herrmann, N., Rapoport, M. J., Rajaram, R. D., Chan, F., Kiss, A., Ma, A. K., . . . Lanctôt, K. L. (2009). Factor analysis of the Rivermead Post-Concussion Symptoms Questionnaire in mild-to-moderate traumatic brain injury patients. *Journal of Neuropsychiatry and Clinical Neurosciences, 21*(2), 181–188.

Heyer, G. L., Young, J. A., Rose, S. C., McNally, K. A., & Fischer, A. N. (2016). Post-traumatic headaches correlate with migraine symptoms in youth with concussion. *Cephalalgia, 36*(4), 309–316. http://dx.doi.org/10.1177/0333102415590240

Hiddema, F. (1963). EEG findings in patients with postconcussion syndrome. *Psychiatria, Neurologia, Neurochirurgia, 66,* 517–521.

Hodges, K., Gordon, Y., & Lennon, M. P. (1990). Parent-child agreement on symptoms assessed via a clinical research interview for children: The Child Assessment Schedule (CAS). *The Journal of Child Psychology and Psychiatry, 31,* 427–436. http://dx.doi.org/10.1111/j.1469-7610.1990.tb01579.x

Hoge, C. W., McGurk, D., Thomas, J. L., Cox, A. L., Engel, C. C., & Castro, C. A. (2008). Mild traumatic brain injury in U.S. soldiers returning from Iraq. *The New England Journal of Medicine, 358,* 453–463. http://dx.doi.org/10.1056/NEJMoa072972

Howell, D. R., O'Brien, M. J., Beasley, M. A., Mannix, R. C., & Meehan, W. P., III. (2016). Initial somatic symptoms are associated with prolonged symptom duration following concussion in adolescents. *Acta Paediatrica, 105,* e426–e432. http://dx.doi.org/10.1111/apa.13486

Howell, D. R., Osternig, L. R., Koester, M. C., & Chou, L. S. (2014). The effect of cognitive task complexity on gait stability in adolescents following concussion. *Experimental Brain Research, 232,* 1773–1782. http://dx.doi.org/10.1007/s00221-014-3869-1

Huang, M. X., Nichols, S., Robb, A., Angeles, A., Drake, A., Holland, M., . . . Lee, R. R. (2012). An automatic MEG low-frequency source imaging approach for detecting injuries in mild and moderate TBI patients with blast and non-blast causes. *NeuroImage, 61,* 1067–1082. http://dx.doi.org/10.1016/j.neuroimage.2012.04.029

Huang, M. X., Theilmann, R. J., Robb, A., Angeles, A., Nichols, S., Drake, A., . . . Lee, R. R. (2009). Integrated imaging approach with MEG and DTI to detect mild traumatic brain injury in military and civilian patients. *Journal of Neurotrauma, 26,* 1213–1226. http://dx.doi.org/10.1089/neu.2008.0672

Hunt, T. N., Ferrara, M. S., Bornstein, R. A., & Baumgartner, T. A. (2009). The reliability of the modified Balance Error Scoring System. *Clinical Journal of Sport Medicine, 19,* 471–475. http://dx.doi.org/10.1097/JSM.0b013e3181c12c7b

Huppert, T. J., Hoge, R. D., Diamond, S. G., Franceschini, M. A., & Boas, D. A. (2006). A temporal comparison of BOLD, ASL, and NIRS hemodynamic responses to motor stimuli in adult humans. *NeuroImage, 29*, 368–382. http://dx.doi.org/10.1016/j.neuroimage.2005.08.065

Ingersoll, C. D., & Armstrong, C. W. (1992). The effects of closed-head injury on postural sway. *Medicine and Science in Sports and Exercise, 24*, 739–743. http://dx.doi.org/10.1249/00005768-199207000-00001

Institute of Medicine, & National Research Council. (2014). *Sports-related concussions in youth: Improving the science, changing the culture.* Washington, DC: The National Academies Press.

Ip, E. Y., Giza, C. C., Griesbach, G. S., & Hovda, D. A. (2002). Effects of enriched environment and fluid percussion injury on dendritic arborization within the cerebral cortex of the developing rat. *Journal of Neurotrauma, 19*, 573–585. http://dx.doi.org/10.1089/089771502753754055

Iverson, G. L. (2006). Misdiagnosis of the persistent postconcussion syndrome in patients with depression. *Archives of Clinical Neuropsychology, 21*, 303–310. http://dx.doi.org/10.1016/j.acn.2005.12.008

Iverson, G. L., Gaetz, M., Lovell, M. R., & Collins, M. W. (2004). Cumulative effects of concussion in amateur athletes. *Brain Injury, 18*, 433–443. http://dx.doi.org/10.1080/02699050310001617352

Iverson, G. L., Gardner, A. J., McCrory, P., Zafonte, R., & Castellani, R. J. (2015). A critical review of chronic traumatic encephalopathy. *Neuroscience and Biobehavioral Reviews, 56*, 276–293. http://dx.doi.org/10.1016/j.neubiorev.2015.05.008

Iverson, G. L., & Lange, R. T. (2003). Examination of "postconcussion-like" symptoms in a healthy sample. *Applied Neuropsychology, 10*(3), 137–144. http://dx.doi.org/10.1207/S15324826AN1003_02

Iverson, G. L., & Schatz, P. (2015). Advanced topics in neuropsychological assessment following sport-related concussion. *Brain Injury, 29*, 263–275. http://dx.doi.org/10.3109/02699052.2014.965214

Jan, J. E., Reiter, R. J., Bax, M. C., Ribary, U., Freeman, R. D., & Wasdell, M. B. (2010). Long-term sleep disturbances in children: A cause of neuronal loss. *European Journal of Paediatric Neurology, 14*, 380–390. http://dx.doi.org/10.1016/j.ejpn.2010.05.001

Janssen, I. (2015). Hyper-parenting is negatively associated with physical activity among 7–12 year olds. *Preventive Medicine, 73*, 55–59. http://dx.doi.org/10.1016/j.ypmed.2015.01.015

Jennett, B., & Bond, M. (1975). Assessment of outcome after severe brain damage. *The Lancet, 1*(7905), 480–484.

Jordan, B. D., Relkin, N. R., Ravdin, L. D., Jacobs, A. R., Bennett, A., & Gandy, S. (1997). Apolipoprotein E epsilon4 associated with chronic traumatic brain injury in boxing. *Journal of the American Medical Association, 278*(2), 136–140. http://dx.doi.org/10.1001/jama.1997.03550020068040

Jorge, R., & Robinson, R. G. (2002). Mood disorders following traumatic brain injury. *NeuroRehabilitation, 17*, 311–324.

Kabat-Zinn, J., Massion, A. O., Kristeller, J., Peterson, L. G., Fletcher, K. E., Pbert, L., . . . Santorelli, S. F. (1992). Effectiveness of a meditation-based stress reduction program in the treatment of anxiety disorders. *The American Journal of Psychiatry, 149*, 936–943. http://dx.doi.org/10.1176/ajp.149.7.936

Kabat-Zinn, J., Wheeler, E., Light, T., Skillings, A., Scharf, M. J., Cropley, T. G., . . . Bernhard, J. D. (1998). Influence of a mindfulness meditation-based stress reduction intervention on rates of skin clearing in patients with moderate to severe psoriasis undergoing phototherapy (UVB) and photochemotherapy (PUVA). *Psychosomatic Medicine, 60*, 625–632. http://dx.doi.org/10.1097/00006842-199809000-00020

Kaminski, T. W., Cousino, E. S., & Glutting, J. J. (2008). Examining the relationship between purposeful heading in soccer and computerized neuropsychological test performance. *Research Quarterly for Exercise and Sport, 79*, 235–244. http://dx.doi.org/10.1080/02701367.2008.10599486

Kashluba, S., Paniak, C., Blake, T., Reynolds, S., Toller-Lobe, G., & Nagy, J. (2004). A longitudinal, controlled study of patient complaints following treated mild traumatic brain injury. *Archives of Clinical Neuropsychology, 19*, 805–816. http://dx.doi.org/10.1016/j.acn.2003.09.005

Kelly, J. P. (2001). Loss of consciousness: Pathophysiology and implications in grading and safe return to play. *Journal of Athletic Training, 36*(3), 249–252.

Kelly, J. P., & Rosenberg, J. H. (1997). Diagnosis and management of concussion in sports. *Neurology, 48*, 575–580. http://dx.doi.org/10.1212/WNL.48.3.575

King, D., Hume, P., Gissane, C., & Clark, T. (2015). Use of the King-Devick test for sideline concussion screening in junior rugby league. *Journal of the Neurological Sciences, 357*, 75–79. http://dx.doi.org/10.1016/j.jns.2015.06.069

King, N. S., Crawford, S., Wenden, F. J., Moss, N. E., & Wade, D. T. (1995). The Rivermead Post Concussion Symptoms Questionnaire: A measure of symptoms commonly experienced after head injury and its reliability. *Journal of Neurology, 242*, 587–592.

Kinnaman, K. A., Mannix, R. C., Comstock, R. D., & Meehan, W. P., III. (2013). Management strategies and medication use for treating paediatric patients with concussions. *Acta Paediatrica, 102*(9), e424–e428. http://dx.doi.org/10.1111/apa.12315

Kochanek, P. M., Bramlett, H. M., Shear, D. A., Dixon, C. E., Mondello, S., Dietrich, W. D., . . . Tortella, F. C. (2016). Synthesis of findings, current investigations, and future directions: Operation brain trauma therapy. *Journal of Neurotrauma, 33*, 606–614. http://dx.doi.org/10.1089/neu.2015.4133

Kontos, A. P., Braithwaite, R., Chrisman, S. P., McAllister-Deitrick, J., Symington, L., Reeves, V., & Collins, M. (2017). Systematic review and meta-analysis of the effects of football heading. *British Journal of Sports Medicine, 51*, 1118–1124. http://dx.doi.org/10.1136/bjsports-2016-096276

Kontos, A. P., Braithwaite, R., Dakan, S., & Elbin, R. J. (2014). Computerized neurocognitive testing and sport-related concussion: Meta-analytic review and analysis of moderating factors within 1 week of injury. *Journal of the International Neuropsychological Society, 20,* 324–332.

Kontos, A. P., Collins, M. W., & Russo, S. (2004). An introduction to sports concussion for the sport psychology consultant. *Journal of Applied Sport Psychology, 16,* 220–235. http://dx.doi.org/10.1080/10413200490485568

Kontos, A. P., Covassin, T., Elbin, R. J., & Parker, T. (2012). Depression and neurocognitive performance after concussion among male and female high school and collegiate athletes. *Archives of Physical Medicine and Rehabilitation, 93,* 1751–1756. http://dx.doi.org/10.1016/j.apmr.2012.03.032

Kontos, A. P., Deitrick, J. M., & Reynolds, E. (2016). Mental health implications and consequences following sport-related concussion. *British Journal of Sports Medicine, 50,* 139–140. http://dx.doi.org/10.1136/bjsports-2015-095564

Kontos, A. P., Dolese, A., Elbin, R. J., Covassin, T., & Warren, B. L. (2011). Relationship of soccer heading to computerized neurocognitive performance and symptoms among female and male youth soccer players. *Brain Injury, 25,* 1234–1241.

Kontos, A. P., & Elbin, R. J. (2013, June). *The cutting edge of concussion research: From the field and lab to the clinic.* Plenary lecture presented at Emerging Frontiers in Concussion: Advancements in Assessment, Management and Rehabilitation, Pittsburgh, PA.

Kontos, A. P., & Elbin, R. J. (2016). Sport-related concussion. In R. Schinke, K. McGannon, & B. Smith (Eds.), *Routledge International handbook of sport psychology* (pp. 204–215). New York, NY: Routledge.

Kontos, A. P., Elbin, R. J., & Collins, M. W. (2006). Aerobic fitness and concussion outcomes in high school football. In S. M. Slobounov & W. J. Sebastianelli (Eds.), *Foundations of sport related brain injuries* (pp. 315–340). New York, NY: Springer.

Kontos, A. P., Elbin, R. J., III, Covassin, T., & Larson, E. (2010). Exploring differences in computerized neurocognitive concussion testing between African American and White athletes. *Archives of Clinical Neuropsychology, 25,* 734–744. http://dx.doi.org/10.1093/arclin/acq068

Kontos, A. P., Elbin, R. J., Kotwal, R., Lutz, R., Kane, S., Benson, P., . . . Collins, M. (2015). The effects of combat-related mild traumatic brain injury (mTBI): Does blast mTBI history matter? *The Journal of Trauma and Acute Care Surgery, 79,* S146–S151.

Kontos, A. P., Elbin, R. J., Lau, B., Simensky, S., Freund, B., French, J., & Collins, M. W. (2013). Posttraumatic migraine as a predictor of recovery and cognitive impairment after sport-related concussion. *The American Journal of Sports Medicine, 41,* 1497–1504. http://dx.doi.org/10.1177/0363546513488751

Kontos, A. P., Elbin, R. J., Newcomer Appaneal, R., Covassin, T., & Collins, M. W. (2013). A comparison of coping responses among high school and college athletes with concussion, orthopedic injuries, and healthy controls. *Research in Sports Medicine, 21,* 367–379.

Kontos, A. P., Elbin, R. J., Schatz, P., Covassin, T., Henry, L., Pardini, J., & Collins, M. W. (2012). A revised factor structure for the Post-Concussion Symptom Scale: Baseline and postconcussion factors. *The American Journal of Sports Medicine, 40,* 2375–2384. http://dx.doi.org/10.1177/0363546512455400

Kontos, A. P., Elbin, R. J., Sufrinko, A., Dakan, S., Bookwalter, K., Price, A., . . . Collins, M. (2016). Incidence of concussion in youth ice hockey players. *Pediatrics, 137*(2), 1–6. http://dx.doi.org/10.1542/peds.2015-1633

Kontos, A. P., Huppert, T. J., Beluk, N. H., Elbin, R. J., Henry, L. C., French, J., . . . Collins, M. W. (2014). Brain activation during neurocognitive testing using functional near-infrared spectroscopy in patients following concussion compared to healthy controls. *Brain Imaging and Behavior, 8,* 621–634. http://dx.doi.org/10.1007/s11682-014-9289-9

Kontos, A. P., Kotwal, R. S., Elbin, R. J., Lutz, R. H., Forsten, R. D., Benson, P. J., & Guskiewicz, K. M. (2013). Residual effects of combat-related mild traumatic brain injury. *Journal of Neurotrauma, 30,* 680–686. http://dx.doi.org/10.1089/neu.2012.2506

Kontos, A. P., McAllister-Deitrick, J., & Reynolds, E. (2016). Mental health implications and consequences following sport-related concussion. *British Journal of Sports Medicine, 50,* 139–140.

Kontos, A. P., & Ortega, J. (2011). Neuromotor effects of concussion: A biobehavioral model. In Frank Webbe (Ed.), *Handbook of sport neuropsychology* (1st ed., pp. 325–326). New York, NY: Springer.

Kontos, A. P., Reches, A., Elbin, R., Dickman, D., Laufer, I., Geva, A., . . . Collins, M. (2016). Preliminary evidence of reduced brain network activation in patients with post traumatic migraine following concussion. *Brian Imaging and Behavior, 10,* 594–603.

Kontos, A. P., Sufrinko, A., Elbin, R. J., Puskar, A., & Collins, M. W. (2016). Reliability and associated risk factors for performance on the Vestibular/Ocular Motor Screening (VOMS) Tool in healthy collegiate athletes. *The American Journal of Sports Medicine, 44,* 1400–1406. http://dx.doi.org/10.1177/0363546516632754

Kontos, A. P., Sufrinko, A., Womble, M., & Kegel, N. (2016). Neuropsychological assessment following concussion: An evidence-based review of the role of neuropsychological assessment pre- and post-concussion. *Current Pain and Headache Reports, 20*(6), 38. http://dx.doi.org/10.1007/s11916-016-0571-y

Kontos, A. P., Van Cott, A. C., Roberts, J., Pan, J. W., Kelly, M. B., McAllister-Deitrick, J., & Hetherington, H. P. (2017). Clinical and magnetic resonance spectroscopic imaging findings in veterans with blast mild traumatic brain injury and post-traumatic stress disorder. *Military Medicine, 182,* 99–104.

Kontos, A. P., Woolford, J., McAllister-Deitrick, J., Sparto, P., Collins, M. W., & Furman, J. (2016). Utility of an incongruent visual, cognitive-balance dual task to assess impairment in athletes with concussion: 3556 June 4, 9:45 AM–10:00 AM. *Medicine and Science in Sports and Exercise, 48*(5, Suppl. 1), 985. http://dx.doi.org/10.1249/01.mss.0000487960.25488.fb

Kostyun, R. O. (2015). Sleep disturbances in concussed athletes: A review of the literature. *Connecticut Medicine, 79,* 161–165.

Kostyun, R. O., & Hafeez, I. (2015). Protracted recovery from a concussion: A focus on gender and treatment interventions in an adolescent population. *Sports Health, 7,* 52–57.

Kostyun, R. O., Milewski, M. D., & Hafeez, I. (2015). Sleep disturbance and neurocognitive function during the recovery from a sport-related concussion in adolescents. *The American Journal of Sports Medicine, 43,* 633–640. http://dx.doi.org/10.1177/0363546514560727

Kovesdi, E., Gyorgy, A. B., Kwon, S. K., Wingo, D. L., Kamnaksh, A., Long, J. B., . . . Agoston, D. V. (2011). The effect of enriched environment on the outcome of traumatic brain injury; A behavioral, proteomics, and histological study. *Frontiers in Neuroscience, 5,* 42. http://dx.doi.org/10.3389/fnins.2011.00042

Kozlowski, K. F., Graham, J., Leddy, J. J., Devinney-Boymel, L., & Willer, B. S. (2013). Exercise intolerance in individuals with postconcussion syndrome. *Journal of Athletic Training, 48,* 627–635. http://dx.doi.org/10.4085/1062-6050-48.5.02

Kristman, V. L., Tator, C. H., Kreiger, N., Richards, D., Mainwaring, L., Jaglal, S., . . . Comper, P. (2008). Does the apolipoprotein-e4 allele predispose varsity athletes to concussion? A prospective cohort study. *Clinical Journal of Sport Medicine, 18,* 322–328.

Kroenke, K., Spitzer, R. L., & Williams, J. B. W. (2001). The PHQ-9: Validity of a brief depression measure. *Journal of General Internal Medicine, 16,* 606–613.

Kuhn, A. W., & Solomon, G. S. (2014). Supervision and computerized neurocognitive baseline test performance in high school athletes: An initial investigation. *Journal of Athletic Training, 49,* 800–805. http://dx.doi.org/10.4085/1062-6050-49.3.66

Kurowski, B. G., Wade, S. L., Dexheimer, J. W., Dyas, J., Zhang, N., & Babcock, L. (2016). Feasibility and potential benefits of a web-based intervention delivered acutely after mild traumatic brain injury in adolescent: A pilot study. *The Journal of Head Trauma and Rehabilitation, 31,* 369–378.

Kwan, V. S., Wojcik, S. P., Miron-Shatz, T., Votruba, A. M., & Olivola, C. Y. (2012). Effects of symptom presentation order on perceived disease risk. *Psychological Science, 23,* 381–385. http://dx.doi.org/10.1177/0956797611432177

Lange, R. T., Panenka, W. J., Shewchuk, J. R., Heran, M. K., Brubacher, J. R., Bioux, S., . . . Iverson, G. L. (2015). Diffusion tensor imaging findings and postconcussion symptom reporting six weeks following mild traumatic brain injury. *Archives of Clinical Neuropsychology, 30*(1), 7–25. http://dx.doi.org/10.1093/arclin/acu060

Langlois, J. A., Rutland-Brown, W., & Wald, M. M. (2006). The epidemiology and impact of traumatic brain injury: A brief overview. *The Journal of Head Trauma Rehabilitation, 21,* 375–378. http://dx.doi.org/10.1097/00001199-200609000-00001

Lau, B. C., Collins, M. W., & Lovell, M. R. (2011). Sensitivity and specificity of subacute computerized neurocognitive testing and symptom evaluation in predicting outcomes after sports-related concussion. *The American Journal of Sports Medicine, 39,* 1209–1216. http://dx.doi.org/10.1177/0363546510392016

Lau, B. C., Collins, M. W., & Lovell, M. R. (2012). Cutoff scores in neurocognitive testing and symptom clusters that predict protracted recovery from concussions in high school athletes. *Neurosurgery, 70,* 371–379. http://dx.doi.org/10.1227/NEU.0b013e31823150f0

Lau, B. C., Kontos, A. P., Collins, M. W., Mucha, A., & Lovell, M. R. (2011). Which on-field signs/symptoms predict protracted recovery from sport-related concussion among high school football players? *The American Journal of Sports Medicine, 39,* 2311–2318. http://dx.doi.org/10.1177/0363546511410655

Lau, B. C., Lovell, M. R., Collins, M. W., & Pardini, J. (2009). Neurocognitive and symptom predictors of recovery in high school athletes. *Clinical Journal of Sport Medicine, 19,* 216–221. http://dx.doi.org/10.1097/JSM.0b013e31819d6edb

Leddy, J. J., Baker, J. G., Kozlowski, K., Bisson, L., & Willer, B. (2011). Reliability of a graded exercise test for assessing recovery from concussion. *Clinical Journal of Sport Medicine, 21*(2), 89–94. http://dx.doi.org/10.1097/JSM.0b013e3181fdc721

Leddy, J. J., Baker, J. G., & Willer, B. (2016). Active rehabilitation of concussion and post-concussion syndrome. *Physical Medicine and Rehabilitation Clinics of North America, 27,* 437–454. http://dx.doi.org/10.1016/j.pmr.2015.12.003

Leddy, J. J., Kozlowski, K., Donnelly, J. P., Pendergast, D. R., Epstein, L. H., & Willer, B. (2010). A preliminary study of subsymptom threshold exercise training for refractory post-concussion syndrome. *Clinical Journal of Sport Medicine, 20*(1), 21–27. http://dx.doi.org/10.1097/JSM.0b013e3181c6c22c

Leddy, J. J., Sandhu, H., Sodhi, V., Baker, J. G., & Willer, B. (2012). Rehabilitation of concussion and post-concussion syndrome. *Sports Health, 4*(2), 147–154. http://dx.doi.org/10.1177/1941738111433673

Leddy, J. J., & Willer, B. (2013). Use of graded exercise testing in concussion and return-to-activity management. *Current Sports Medicine Reports, 12,* 370–376. http://dx.doi.org/10.1249/JSR.0000000000000008

Lee, R. R., & Huang, M. (2014). Magnetoencephalography in the diagnosis of concussion. *Progress in Neurological Surgery, 28,* 94–111. http://dx.doi.org/10.1159/000358768

Leslie, O., & Craton, N. (2013). Concussion: Purely a brain injury? *Clinical Journal of Sport Medicine, 23,* 331–332. http://dx.doi.org/10.1097/JSM.0b013e318295bbb1

Levinson, D. M., & Reeves, D. L. (1997). Monitoring recovery from traumatic brain injury using Automated Neuropsychological Assessment Metrics (ANAM V1.0). *Archives of Clinical Neuropsychology, 12,* 155–166.

Lew, H. L., Vanderploeg, R. D., Moore, D. F., Schwab, K., Friedman, L., Yesavage, J., . . . Sigford, B. J. (2008). Overlap of mild TBI and mental health conditions in returning OIF/OEF service members and veterans. *Journal of Rehabilitation Research and Development, 45*(3), xi–xvi.

Lewine, J. D., Davis, J. T., Bigler, E. D., Thoma, R., Hill, D., Funke, M., . . . Orrison, W. W. (2007). Objective documentation of traumatic brain injury subsequent to mild head trauma: Multimodal brain imaging with MEG, SPECT, and MRI. *The Journal of Head Trauma Rehabilitation, 22*(3), 141–155. http://dx.doi.org/10.1097/01.HTR.0000271115.29954.27

Lincoln, A. E., Caswell, S. V., Almquist, J. L., Dunn, R. E., Norris, J. B., & Hinton, R. Y. (2011). Trends in concussion incidence in high school sports: A prospective 11-year study. *The American Journal of Sports Medicine, 39,* 958–963. http://dx.doi.org/10.1177/0363546510392326

Lipton, M. L., Gellella, E., Lo, C., Gold, T., Ardekani, B. A., Shifteh, K., . . . Branch, C. A. (2008). Multifocal white matter ultrastructural abnormalities in mild traumatic brain injury with cognitive disability: A voxel-wise analysis of diffusion tensor imaging. *Journal of Neurotrauma, 25,* 1335–1342. http://dx.doi.org/10.1089/neu.2008.0547

Love, S., & Solomon, G. S. (2015). Talking with parents of high school football players about chronic traumatic encephalopathy: A concise summary. *The American Journal of Sports Medicine, 43,* 1260–1264. http://dx.doi.org/10.1177/0363546514535187

Lovell, M. R., & Collins, M. W. (1998). Neuropsychological assessment of the college football player. *The Journal of Head Trauma Rehabilitation, 13*(2), 9–26. http://dx.doi.org/10.1097/00001199-199804000-00004

Lovell, M. R., Iverson, G. L., Collins, M. W., McKeag, D., & Maroon, J. C. (1999). Does loss of consciousness predict neuropsychological decrements after concussion? *Clinical Journal of Sport Medicine, 9*(4), 193–198. http://dx.doi.org/10.1097/00042752-199910000-00002

Lovell, M. R., Iverson, G. L., Collins, M. W., Podell, K., Johnston, K. M., Pardini, D., . . . Maroon, J. C. (2006). Measurement of symptoms following sports-related concussion: Reliability and normative data for the post-concussion scale. *Applied Neuropsychology, 13*(3), 166–174.

Lovell, M. R., Pardini, J. E., Welling, J., Collins, M. W., Bakal, J., Lazar, N., . . . Becker, J. T. (2007). Functional brain abnormalities are related to clinical recovery and time to return-to-play in athletes. *Neurosurgery, 61,* 352–359. http://dx.doi.org/10.1227/01.NEU.0000279985.94168.7F

MacDonald, C. L., Johnson, A. M., Wierzechowski, L., Kassner, E., Stewart, T., Nelson, E. C., . . . Brody, D. L. (2014). Prospectively assessed clinical outcomes in concussive blast vs nonblast traumatic brain injury among evacuated US military personnel. *JAMA Neurology, 71,* 994–1002.

Maerlender, A., Rieman, W., Lichtenstein, J., & Condiracci, C. (2015). Programmed physical exertion in recovery from sports-related concussion: A randomized pilot study. *Developmental Neuropsychology, 40*(5), 273–278. http://dx.doi.org/10.1080/87565641.2015.1067706

Maher, M. E., Hutchison, M., Cusimano, M., Comper, P., & Schweizer, T. A. (2014). Concussions and heading in soccer: A review of the evidence of incidence, mechanisms, biomarkers and neurocognitive outcomes. *Brain Injury, 28*(3), 271–285. http://dx.doi.org/10.3109/02699052.2013.865269

Mainwaring, L. M., Bisschop, S., Green, R. E. A., Antoniazzi, M., Comper, P., Kristman, V., . . . Richards, D. W. (2004). Emotional reaction of varsity athletes to sport-related concussion. *Journal of Sport & Exercise Psychology, 26*, 119–135. http://dx.doi.org/10.1123/jsep.26.1.119

Mainwaring, L. M., Hutchison, M., Bisschop, S. M., Comper, P., & Richards, D. W. (2010). Emotional response to sport concussion compared to ACL injury. *Brain Injury, 24*, 589–597. http://dx.doi.org/10.3109/02699051003610508

Majerske, C. W., Mihalik, J. P., Ren, D., Collins, M. W., Reddy, C. C., Lovell, M. R., & Wagner, A. K. (2008). Concussion in sports: Postconcussive activity levels, symptoms, and neurocognitive performance. *Journal of Athletic Training, 43*(3), 265–274. http://dx.doi.org/10.4085/1062-6050-43.3.265

Manners, J. L., Forsten, R. D., Kotwal, R. S., Elbin, R. J., Collins, M. W., & Kontos, A. P. (2016). Role of pre-morbid factors and exposure to blast mild traumatic brain injury on post-traumatic stress in United States military personnel. *Journal of Neurotrauma, 33*, 1796–1801. http://dx.doi.org/10.1089/neu.2015.4245

Matser, J. T., Kessels, A. G., Jordan, B. D., Lezak, M. D., & Troost, J. (1998). Chronic traumatic brain injury in professional soccer players. *Neurology, 51*, 791–796. http://dx.doi.org/10.1212/WNL.51.3.791

Mayer, A. R., Ling, J., Mannell, M. V., Gasparovic, C., Phillips, J. P., Doezema, D., . . . Yeo, R. A. (2010). A prospective diffusion tensor imaging study in mild traumatic brain injury. *Neurology, 74*, 643–650. http://dx.doi.org/10.1212/WNL.0b013e3181d0ccdd

Mayers, L. B., & Redick, T. S. (2012). Clinical utility of ImPACT assessment for postconcussion return-to-play counseling: Psychometric issues. *Journal of Clinical and Experimental Neuropsychology, 34*, 235–242. http://dx.doi.org/10.1080/13803395.2011.630655

McAvoy, K. (2009). *REAP the benefits of good concussion management: How every school, parent and doctor can create a community-based concussion management program.* Denver, CO: Brain Injury Team, Cherry Creek School District.

McCaffrey, M. A., Mihalik, J. P., Crowell, D. H., Shields, E. W., & Guskiewicz, K. M. (2007). Measurement of head impacts in collegiate football players: Clinical measures of concussion after high- and low-magnitude impacts. *Neurosurgery, 61*, 1236–1243. http://dx.doi.org/10.1227/01.neu.0000306102.91506.8b

McClure, D. J., Zuckerman, S. L., Kutscher, S. J., Gregory, A. J., & Solomon, G. S. (2014). Baseline neurocognitive testing in sports-related concussions: The importance of a prior night's sleep. *The American Journal of Sports Medicine, 42*, 472–478. http://dx.doi.org/10.1177/0363546513510389

McCrae, R. R., & Costa, P. T., Jr. (2004). A contemplated revision of the NEO Five-Factor Inventory. *Personality and Individual Differences, 36*, 587–596.

McCrea, M., Guskiewicz, K. M., Marshall, S. W., Barr, W., Randolph, C., Cantu, R. C., . . . Kelly, J. P. (2003). Acute effects and recovery time following concussion in collegiate football players: The NCAA concussion study. *Journal of the American Medical Association, 290,* 2556–2563.

McCrea, M., Guskiewicz, K., Randolph, C., Barr, W. B., Hammeke, T. A., Marshall, S. W., . . . Kelly, J. P. (2013). Incidence, clinical course, and predictors of prolonged recovery time following sport-related concussion in high school and college athletes. *Journal of the International Neuropsychological Society, 19*(1), 22–33. http://dx.doi.org/10.1017/S1355617712000872

McCrea, M., Kelly, J. P., Randolph, C., Kluge, J., Bartolic, E., Finn, G., & Baxter, B. (1998). Standardized assessment of concussion (SAC): On-site mental status evaluation of the athlete. *Journal of Head Trauma Rehabilitation, 13*(2), 27–35.

McCrea, M., Prichep, L., Powell, M. R., Chabot, R., & Barr, W. B. (2010). Acute effects and recovery after sport-related concussion: A neurocognitive and quantitative brain electrical activity study. *The Journal of Head Trauma Rehabilitation, 25,* 283–292. http://dx.doi.org/10.1097/HTR.0b013e3181e67923

McCrory, P. R., & Berkovic, S. F. (2001). Concussion: The history of clinical and pathophysiological concepts and misconceptions. *Neurology, 57,* 2283–2289. http://dx.doi.org/10.1212/WNL.57.12.2283

McCrory, P. R., Davis, G., & Makdissi, M. (2012). Second impact syndrome or cerebral swelling after sporting head injury. *Current Sports Medicine Reports, 11*(1), 21–23. http://dx.doi.org/10.1249/JSR.0b013e3182423bfd

McCrory, P. R., Johnston, K., Meeuwisse, W., Aubry, M., Cantu, R., Dvořák, J., . . . Schamasch, P. (2005). Summary and agreement statement of the second international conference on concussion in sport, Prague 2004. *The Physician and Sportsmedicine, 33*(4), 29–44. http://dx.doi.org/10.3810/psm.2005.04.76

McCrory, P. R., Meeuwisse, W., Aubry, M., Cantu, B., Dvořák, J., Echemendia, R., . . . Turner, M. (2013). Consensus statement on Concussion in Sport—The 4th International Conference on Concussion in Sport held in Zurich, November 2012. *Physical Therapy in Sport, 14,* e1–e13. http://dx.doi.org/10.1016/j.ptsp.2013.03.002

McCrory, P. R., Meeuwisse, W., Dvořák, J., Aubry, M., Bailes, J., Broglio, S., . . . Vos, P. E. (2017). Consensus statement on concussion in sport—The 5th international conference on concussion in sport held in Berlin, October 2016. *British Journal of Sports Medicine.* Retrieved from http://bjsm.bmj.com/content/early/2017/04/28/bjsports-2017-097699

McCrory, P. R., Meeuwisse, W., Johnston, K., Dvořák, J., Aubry, M., Molloy, M., & Cantu, R. (2009). Consensus statement on concussion in sport—the Third International Conference on Concussion in Sport held in Zurich, November 2008. *The Physician and Sportsmedicine, 37,* 141–159. http://dx.doi.org/10.3810/psm.2009.06.1721

McGrath, N., Dinn, W. M., Collins, M. W., Lovell, M. R., Elbin, R. J., & Kontos, A. P. (2013). Post-exertion neurocognitive test failure among student-athletes following concussion. *Brain Injury, 27*(1), 103–113. http://dx.doi.org/10.3109/02699052.2012.729282

McKee, A. C., Cairns, N. J., Dickson, D. W., Folkerth, R. D., Keene, C. D., Litvan, I., . . . TBI/CTE Group. (2016). The first NINDS/NIBIB consensus meeting to define neuropathological criteria for the diagnosis of chronic traumatic encephalopathy. *Acta Neuropathologica, 131*, 75–86.

McKee, A. C., Cantu, R. C., Nowinski, C. J., Hedley-Whyte, E. T., Gavett, B. E., Budson, A. E., . . . Stern, R. A. (2009). Chronic traumatic encephalopathy in athletes: Progressive tauopathy after repetitive head injury. *Journal of Neuropathology and Experimental Neurology, 68*, 709–735. http://dx.doi.org/10.1097/NEN.0b013e3181a9d503

McLendon, L. A., Kralik, S. F., Grayson, P. A., & Golomb, M. R. (2016). The controversial second impact syndrome: A review of the literature. *Pediatric Neurology, 62*, 9–17. http://dx.doi.org/10.1016/j.pediatrneurol.2016.03.009

McMillan, T. J., Robertson, I. H., Brock, D., & Chorlton, L. (2002). Brief mindfulness training for attentional problems after traumatic brain injury: A randomised control treatment trial. *Neuropsychological Rehabilitation, 12*(2), 117–125. http://dx.doi.org/10.1080/09602010143000202

McNair, P. M., Lorr, M., & Droppleman, L. F. (1981). *POMS manual* (2nd ed.). San Diego, CA: Educational and Industrial Testing Service.

Meehan, W. P., III. (2011). Medical therapies for concussion. *Clinics in Sports Medicine, 30*(1), 115–124. http://dx.doi.org/10.1016/j.csm.2010.08.003

Meehan, W. P., III, Mannix, R. C., Stracciolini, A., Elbin, R. J., & Collins, M. W. (2013). Symptom severity predicts prolonged recovery after sport-related concussion, but age and amnesia do not. *The Journal of Pediatrics, 163*, 721–725. http://dx.doi.org/10.1016/j.jpeds.2013.03.012

Meehan, W. P., III, Taylor, A. M., & Proctor, M. (2011). The pediatric athlete: Younger athletes with sport-related concussion. *Clinics in Sports Medicine, 30*(1), 133–144. http://dx.doi.org/10.1016/j.csm.2010.08.004

Meier, T. B., Bellgowan, P. S., Singh, R., Kuplicki, R., Polanski, D. W., & Mayer, A. R. (2015). Recovery of cerebral blood flow following sports-related concussion. *JAMA Neurology, 72*, 530–538. http://dx.doi.org/10.1001/jamaneurol.2014.4778

Mendez, M. F., Owens, E. M., Reza Berenji, G., Peppers, D. C., Liang, L. J., & Licht, E. A. (2013). Mild traumatic brain injury from primary blast vs. blunt forces: Post-concussion consequences and functional neuroimaging. *NeuroRehabilitation, 32*(2), 397–407.

Merritt, V. C., & Arnett, P. A. (2014). Premorbid predictors of postconcussion symptoms in collegiate athletes. *Journal of Clinical and Experimental Neuropsychology, 36*, 1098–1111. http://dx.doi.org/10.1080/13803395.2014.983463

Merritt, V. C., Rabinowitz, A. R., & Arnett, P. A. (2015). Personality factors and symptom reporting at baseline in collegiate athletes. *Developmental Neuropsychology, 40*, 45–50.

Mihalik, J. P., Lengas, E., Register-Mihalik, J. K., Oyama, S., Begalle, R. L., & Guskiewicz, K. M. (2013). The effects of sleep quality and sleep quantity on concussion baseline assessment. *Clinical Journal of Sport Medicine, 23*, 343–348. http://dx.doi.org/10.1097/JSM.0b013e318295a834

Mihalik, J. P., Stump, J. E., Collins, M. W., Lovell, M. R., Field, M., & Maroon, J. C. (2005). Posttraumatic migraine characteristics in athletes following sports-related concussion. *Journal of Neurosurgery, 102*, 850–855. http://dx.doi.org/10.3171/jns.2005.102.5.0850

Miles, L., Grossman, R. I., Johnson, G., Babb, J. S., Diller, L., & Inglese, M. (2008). Short-term DTI predictors of cognitive dysfunction in mild traumatic brain injury. *Brain Injury, 22*, 115–122. http://dx.doi.org/10.1080/02699050801888816

Miller, L. S., Colella, B., Mikulis, D., Maller, J., & Green, R. E. (2013). Environmental enrichment may protect against hippocampal atrophy in the chronic stages of traumatic brain injury. *Frontiers in Human Neuroscience, 7*, 506. http://dx.doi.org/10.3389/fnhum.2013.00506

Moldovan, M., Constantinescu, A. O., Balseanu, A., Oprescu, N., Zagrean, L., & Popa-Wagner, A. (2010). Sleep deprivation attenuates experimental stroke severity in rats. *Experimental Neurology, 222*, 135–143.

Mondaini, N., Gontero, P., Giubilei, G., Lombardi, G., Cai, T., Gavazzi, A., & Bartoletti, R. (2007). Finasteride 5 mg and sexual side effects: How many of these are related to a nocebo phenomenon? *Journal of Sexual Medicine, 4*, 1708–1712. http://dx.doi.org/10.1111/j.1743-6109.2007.00563.x

Montenigro, P. H., Alosco, M. L., Martin, B. M., Daneshvar, D. H., Mez, J., Chaisson, C. E., . . . Tripodis, Y. (2017). Cumulative head impact exposure predicts later-life depression, apathy, executive dysfunction, and cognitive impairment in former high school and college football players. *Journal of Neurotrauma, 34*, 328–340.

Montenigro, P. H., Bernick, C., & Cantu, R. C. (2015). Clinical features of repetitive traumatic brain injury and chronic traumatic encephalopathy. *Brain Pathology, 25*, 304–317. http://dx.doi.org/10.1111/bpa.12250

Morgan, C. D., Zuckerman, S. L., King, L. E., Beaird, S. E., Sills, A. K., & Solomon, G. S. (2015). Post-Concussion Syndrome (PCS) in a youth population: Defining the diagnostic value and cost-utility of brain imaging. *Child's Nervous System, 31*, 2305–2309. http://dx.doi.org/10.1007/s00381-015-2916-y

Mortenson, P., Singhal, A., Hengel, A. R., & Purtzki, J. (2016). Impact of early follow-up intervention on parent-reported postconcussion pediatric symptoms: A feasibility study. *The Journal of Head Trauma Rehabilitation, 31*, E23–E32. http://dx.doi.org/10.1097/HTR.0000000000000223

Moser, R. S., Glatts, C., & Schatz, P. (2012). Efficacy of immediate and delayed cognitive and physical rest for treatment of sports-related concussion. *Journal of Pediatrics, 161*, 922–926.

Moser, R. S., Schatz, P., Neidzwski, K., & Ott, S. D. (2011). Group versus individual administration affects baseline neurocognitive test performance. *The*

American Journal of Sports Medicine, 39, 2325–2330. http://dx.doi.org/10.1177/0363546511417114

Mrazik, M., Brooks, B. L., Jubinville, A., Meeuwisse, W. H., & Emery, C. A. (2016). Psychosocial outcomes of sport concussions in youth hockey players. *Archives of Clinical Neuropsychology, 31*(4), 297–304. http://dx.doi.org/10.1093/arclin/acw013

Mucha, A., Collins, M. W., Elbin, R. J., Furman, J. M., Troutman-Enseki, C., DeWolf, R. M., . . . Kontos, A. P. (2014). A brief Vestibular/Ocular Motor Screening (VOMS) assessment to evaluate concussions: Preliminary findings. *The American Journal of Sports Medicine, 42,* 2479–2486. http://dx.doi.org/10.1177/0363546514543775

Munce, T. A., Dorman, J. C., Thompson, P. A., Valentine, V. D., & Bergeron, M. F. (2015). Head impact exposure and neurologic function of youth football players. *Medicine and Science in Sports and Exercise, 47,* 1567–1576. http://dx.doi.org/10.1249/MSS.0000000000000591

Murray, N., Salvatore, A., Powell, D., & Reed-Jones, R. (2014). Reliability and validity evidence of multiple balance assessments in athletes with a concussion. *Journal of Athletic Training, 49,* 540–549. http://dx.doi.org/10.4085/1062-6050-49.3.32

National Collegiate Athletic Association Sport Science Institute. (2016). *Concussion diagnosis and management: Best practices* [Interassociation consensus document]. Retrieved from http://www.ncaa.org/sport-science-institute/concussion-diagnosis-and-management-best-practices

National Institute of Neurological Disorders and Stroke. (n.d.). *NINDS common data elements.* Retrieved from https://www.commondataelements.ninds.nih.gov/SRC.aspx#tab=Data_Standards

Nelson, L. D., Pfaller, A. Y., Rein, L. E., & McCrea, M. A. (2015). Rates and predictors of invalid baseline test performance in high school and collegiate athletes for three computerized neurocognitive tests (CNTs): ANAM, Axon, and ImPACT. *The American Journal of Sports Medicine, 43,* 2018–2026. http://dx.doi.org/10.1177/0363546515587714

Niogi, S. N., Mukherjee, P., Ghajar, J., Johnson, C., Kolster, R. A., Sarkar, R., . . . McCandliss, B. D. (2008). Extent of microstructural white matter injury in postconcussive syndrome correlates with impaired cognitive reaction time: A 3T diffusion tensor imaging study of mild traumatic brain injury. *American Journal of Neuroradiology, 29,* 967–973. http://dx.doi.org/10.3174/ajnr.A0970

Nithianantharajah, J., & Hannan, A. J. (2006). Enriched environments, experience-dependent plasticity and disorders of the nervous system. *Nature Reviews Neuroscience, 7,* 697–709.

O'Kane, J. W., Spieker, A., Levy, M. R., Neradilek, M., Polissar, N. L., & Schiff, M. A. (2014). Concussion among female middle-school soccer players. *JAMA Pediatrics, 168*(3), 258–264. http://dx.doi.org/10.1001/jamapediatrics.2013.4518

Oldham, J. R., Munkasy, B. A., Evans, K. M., Wikstrom, E. A., & Buckley, T. A. (2016). Altered dynamic postural control during gait termination following concussion. *Gait & Posture, 49*, 437–442. http://dx.doi.org/10.1016/j.gaitpost. 2016.07.327

Omalu, B. I., Hamilton, R. L., Kamboh, M. I., DeKosky, S. T., & Bailes, J. (2010). Chronic traumatic encephalopathy (CTE) in a National Football League player: Case report and emerging medicolegal practice questions. *Journal of Forensic Nursing, 6*(1), 40–46. http://dx.doi.org/10.1111/j.1939-3938.2009.01064.x

O'Neil, M. E., Carlson, K., Storzbach, D., Brenner, L., Freeman, M., Quinones, A., & Kansagara, D. (2013). *Complications of mild traumatic brain injury in veterans and military personnel: A systematic review.* Washington, DC: Department of Veterans Affairs Health Services Research & Development Service.

Paolicelli, R. C., Bolasco, G., Pagani, F., Maggi, L., Scianni, M., Panzanelli, P., . . . Gross, C. T. (2011). Synaptic pruning by microglia is necessary for normal brain development. *Science, 333*(6048), 1456–1458. http://dx.doi.org/10.1126/science.1202529

Papa, L., Brophy, G. M., Welch, R. D., Lewis, L. M., Braga, C. F., Tan, C. N., . . . Hack, D. C. (2016). Time course and diagnostic accuracy of glial and neuronal blood biomarkers GFAP and UCH-L1 in a large cohort of trauma patients with and without mild traumatic brain injury. *JAMA Neurology, 73*, 551–560. http://dx.doi.org/10.1001/jamaneurol.2016.0039

Papa, L., Silvestri, S., Brophy, G. M., Giordano, P., Falk, J. L., Braga, C. F., . . . Robertson, C. S. (2014). GFAP out-performs S100β in detecting traumatic intracranial lesions on computed tomography in trauma patients with mild traumatic brain injury and those with extracranial lesions. *Journal of Neurotrauma, 31*, 1815–1822. http://dx.doi.org/10.1089/neu.2013.3245

Pardini, D., Stump, J., Lovell, M. R., Collins, M. W., Moritz, K., & Fu, F. (2004). The Post-Concussion Symptom Scale (PCSS): A factor analysis. *British Journal of Sports Medicine, 38*, 654–664.

Parmet, S., Lynm, C., & Glass, R. M. (2003). Concussion in sports. *Journal of the American Medical Association, 290*, 2628. http://dx.doi.org/10.1001/jama. 290.19.2520

Pasek, T. A., Locasto, L. W., Reichard, J., Fazio Sumrok, V. C., Johnson, E. W., & Kontos, A. P. (2015). The headache electronic diary for children with concussion. *Clinical Nurse Specialist, 29*(2), 80–88. http://dx.doi.org/10.1097/NUR.0000000000000108

Pearce, K. L., Sufrinko, A., Lau, B. C., Henry, L., Collins, M. W., & Kontos, A. P. (2015). Near point of convergence after a sport-related concussion: Measurement reliability and relationship to neurocognitive impairment and symptoms. *The American Journal of Sports Medicine, 43*, 3055–3061. http://dx.doi.org/10.1177/0363546515606430

Pellman, E. J., Viano, D. C., Tucker, A. M., Casson, I. R., & Committee on Mild Traumatic Brain Injury, National Football League (2003). Concussion in professional football: Location and direction of helmet impacts-Part 2. *Neurosurgery, 53,* 1328–1341.

Petraglia, A. L., Maroon, J. C., & Bailes, J. E. (2012). From the field of play to the field of combat: A review of the pharmacological management of concussion. *Neurosurgery, 70,* 1520–1533. http://dx.doi.org/10.1227/NEU.0b013e31824cebe8

Piland, S. G., Ferrara, M. S., Macciocchi, S. N., Broglio, S. P., & Gould, T. E. (2010). Investigation of baseline self-report concussion symptom scores. *Journal of Athletic Training, 45,* 273–278. http://dx.doi.org/10.4085/1062-6050-45.3.273

Piland, S. G., Motl, R. W., Ferrara, M. S., & Peterson, C. L. (2003). Evidence for the factorial and construct validity of a self-report concussion symptoms scale. *Journal of Athletic Training, 38,* 104–112.

Piland, S. G., Motl, R. W., Guskiewicz, K. M., McCrea, M., & Ferrara, M. S. (2006). Structural validity of a self-report concussion-related symptom scale. *Medicine and Science in Sports and Exercise, 38*(1), 27–32. http://dx.doi.org/10.1249/01.mss.0000183186.98212.d5

Podlog, L., & Eklund, R. C. (2004). Assisting injured athletes with the return to sport transition. *Clinical Journal of Sport Medicine, 14,* 257–259. http://dx.doi.org/10.1097/00042752-200409000-00001

Ponsford, J. L., Ziino, C., Parcell, D. L., Shekleton, J. A., Roper, M., Redman, J. R., . . . Rajaratnam, S. M. (2012). Fatigue and sleep disturbance following traumatic brain injury—their nature, causes, and potential treatments. *The Journal of Head Trauma Rehabilitation, 27,* 224–233. http://dx.doi.org/10.1097/HTR.0b013e31824ee1a8

Presson, N., Beers, S. R., Morrow, L., Wagener, L. M., Bird, W. A., Van Eman, G., . . . Schneider, W. (2015). An exploratory analysis linking neuropsychological testing to quantification of tractography using high definition fiber tracking (HDFT) in military TBI. *Brain Imaging and Behavior, 9,* 484–499. http://dx.doi.org/10.1007/s11682-015-9386-4

Pulsipher, D. T., Campbell, R. A., Thoma, R., & King, J. H. (2011). A critical review of neuroimaging applications in sports concussion. *Current Sports Medicine Reports, 10,* 14–20. http://dx.doi.org/10.1249/JSR.0b013e31820711b8

Purcell, L., Harvey, J., & Seabrook, J. A. (2016). Patterns of recovery following sport-related concussion in children and adolescents. *Clinical Pediatrics, 55,* 452–458. http://dx.doi.org/10.1177/0009922815589915

Putukian, M., Echemendia, R. J., & Mackin, S. (2000). The acute neuropsychological effects of heading in soccer: A pilot study. *Clinical Journal of Sport Medicine, 10,* 104–109. http://dx.doi.org/10.1097/00042752-200004000-00004

Randolph, C. (1998). *RBANS manual: Repeatable battery for the assessment of neuropsychological status.* San Antonio, TX: Psychological Corporation.

Randolph, C. (2011). Baseline neuropsychological testing in managing sport-related concussion: Does it modify risk? *Current Sports Medicine Reports, 10*(1), 21–26. http://dx.doi.org/10.1249/JSR.0b013e318207831d

Randolph, C., Millis, S., Barr, W. B., McCrea, M., Guskiewicz, K. M., Hammeke, T. A., & Kelly, J. P. (2009). Concussion symptom inventory: An empirically derived scale for monitoring resolution of symptoms following sport-related concussion. *Archives of Clinical Neuropsychology, 24*(3), 219–229. http://dx.doi.org/10.1093/arclin/acp025

Ransom, D. M., Vaughan, C. G., Pratson, L., Sady, M. D., McGill, C. A., & Gioia, G. A. (2015). Academic effects of concussion in children and adolescents. *Pediatrics, 135,* 1043–1050. http://dx.doi.org/10.1542/peds.2014-3434

Reddy, C. C., Collins, M., Lovell, M., & Kontos, A. P. (2013). Efficacy of amantadine treatment on symptoms and neurocognitive performance among adolescents following sports-related concussion. *The Journal of Head Trauma Rehabilitation, 28,* 260–265. http://dx.doi.org/10.1097/HTR.0b013e318257fbc6

Reger, M. L., Poulos, A. M., Buen, F., Giza, C. C., Hovda, D. A., & Fanselow, M. S. (2012). Concussive brain injury enhances fear learning and excitatory processes in the amygdala. *Biological Psychiatry, 71,* 335–343. http://dx.doi.org/10.1016/j.biopsych.2011.11.007

Register-Mihalik, J. K., Littleton, A. C., & Guskiewicz, K. M. (2013). Are divided attention tasks useful in the assessment and management of sport-related concussion? *Neuropsychology Review, 23,* 300–313. http://dx.doi.org/10.1007/s11065-013-9238-1

Rey, J. M., Schrader, E., & Morris-Yates, A. (1992). Parent–child agreement on children's behaviours reported by the Child Behaviour Checklist (CBCL). *Journal of Adolescence, 15*(3), 219–230. http://dx.doi.org/10.1016/0140-1971(92)90026-2

Rhine, T., Babcock, L., Zhang, N., Leach, J., & Wade, S. L. (2016). Are UCH-L1 and GFAP promising biomarkers for children with mild traumatic brain injury? *Brain Injury, 30,* 1231–1238. http://dx.doi.org/10.1080/02699052.2016.1178396

Richman, J. M., Rosenfeld, L., & Hardy, C. J. (1993). The Social Support Survey: A validation of a clinical measure of the social support process. *Research on Social Work Practice, 3,* 288–311. http://dx.doi.org/10.1177/104973159300300304

Risling, M., Plantman, S., Angeria, M., Rostami, E., Bellander, B. M., Kirkegaard, M., . . . Davidsson, J. (2011). Mechanisms of blast induced brain injuries, experimental studies in rats. *NeuroImage, 54*(Suppl. 1), S89–S97. http://dx.doi.org/10.1016/j.neuroimage.2010.05.031

Rizzo, J. R., Hudson, T. E., Dai, W., Desai, N., Yousefi, A., Palsana, D., . . . Rucker, J. C. (2016). Objectifying eye movements during rapid number naming: Methodology for assessment of normative data for the King-Devick test. *Journal of the Neurological Sciences, 362,* 232–239. http://dx.doi.org/10.1016/j.jns.2016.01.045

Rogers, J. H. (1980). Romberg and his test. *The Journal of Laryngology and Otology, 94,* 1401–1404. http://dx.doi.org/10.1017/S002221510009023X

Roof, R. L., & Hall, E. D. (2000). Gender differences in acute CNS trauma and stroke: Neuroprotective effects of estrogen and progesterone. *Journal of Neurotrauma, 17,* 367–388. http://dx.doi.org/10.1089/neu.2000.17.367

Root, J. M., Zuckerbraun, N. S., Wang, L., Winger, D. G., Brent, D., Kontos, A., & Hickey, R. W. (2016). History of somatization is associated with prolonged recovery from concussion. *Journal of Pediatrics*, *174*, 39–44. http://dx.doi.org/10.1016/j.jpeds.2016.03.020

Rowhani-Rahbar, A., Chrisman, S. P., Drescher, S., Schiff, M. A., & Rivara, F. P. (2016). Agreement between high school athletes and their parents on reporting athletic events and concussion symptoms. *Journal of Neurotrauma*, *33*(8), 784–791.

Rowson, S., Duma, S. M., Beckwith, J. G., Chu, J. J., Greenwald, R. M., Crisco, J. J., . . . Maerlender, A. C. (2012). Rotational head kinematics in football impacts: An injury risk function for concussion. *Annals of Biomedical Engineering*, *40*(1), 1–13. http://dx.doi.org/10.1007/s10439-011-0392-4

Roy, S., & Irvin, R. (1983). *Sports medicine*. Upper Saddle River, NJ: Prentice Hall.

Ruff, R. M., Crouch, J. A., Tröster, A. I., Marshall, L. F., Buchsbaum, M. S., Lottenberg, S., & Somers, L. M. (1994). Selected cases of poor outcome following a minor brain trauma: Comparing neuropsychological and positron emission tomography assessment. *Brain Injury*, *8*(4), 297–308. http://dx.doi.org/10.3109/02699059409150981

Saatman, K. E., Duhaime, A. C., Bullock, R., Maas, A. I., Valadka, A., Manley, G. T., & the Workshop Scientific Team and Advisory Panel Members. (2008). Classification of traumatic brain injury for targeted therapies. *Journal of Neurotrauma*, *25*, 719–738. http://dx.doi.org/10.1089/neu.2008.0586

Sandel, N. K., Lovell, M. R., Kegel, N. E., Collins, M. W., & Kontos, A. P. (2013). The relationship of symptoms and neurocognitive performance to perceived recovery from sports-related concussion among adolescent athletes. *Applied Neuropsychology: Child*, *2*(1), 64–69. http://dx.doi.org/10.1080/21622965.2012.670580

Sarmiento, K., Hoffman, R., Dmitrovsky, Z., & Lee, R. (2014). A 10-year review of the Centers for Disease Control and Prevention's *Heads Up* initiatives: Bringing concussion awareness to the forefront. *Journal of Safety Research*, *50*, 143–147. http://dx.doi.org/10.1016/j.jsr.2014.05.003

Schaaf, M. J., de Jong, J., de Kloet, E. R., & Vreugdenhil, E. (1998). Downregulation of BDNF mRNA and protein in the rat hippocampus by corticosterone. *Brain Research*, *813*, 112–120. http://dx.doi.org/10.1016/S0006-8993(98)01010-5

Schatz, P., & Glatts, C. (2013). "Sandbagging" baseline test performance on ImPACT, without detection, is more difficult than it appears. *Archives of Clinical Neuropsychology*, *28*, 236–244. http://dx.doi.org/10.1093/arclin/act009

Schatz, P., Moser, R. S., Solomon, G. S., Ott, S. D., & Karpf, R. (2012). Prevalence of invalid computerized baseline neurocognitive test results in high school and collegiate athletes. *Journal of Athletic Training*, *47*, 289–296. http://dx.doi.org/10.4085/1062-6050-47.3.14

Schnadower, D., Vazquez, H., Lee, J., Dayan, P., & Roskind, C. G. (2007). Controversies in the evaluation and management of minor blunt head trauma in children. *Current Opinion in Pediatrics, 19,* 258–264. http://dx.doi.org/10.1097/MOP.0b013e3281084e85

Schnebel, B., Gwin, J. T., Anderson, S., & Gatlin, R. (2007). In vivo study of head impacts in football: A comparison of National Collegiate Athletic Association Division I versus high school impacts. *Neurosurgery, 60,* 490–496. http://dx.doi.org/10.1227/01.NEU.0000249286.92255.7F

Schneider, K. J., Meeuwisse, W. H., Nettel-Aguirre, A., Barlow, K., Boyd, L., Kang, J., & Emery, C. A. (2014). Cervicovestibular rehabilitation in sport-related concussion: A randomised controlled trial. *British Journal of Sports Medicine, 48,* 1294–1298. http://dx.doi.org/10.1136/bjsports-2013-093267

Schneider, W., Okonkwo, D. O., Presson, N., Marrow, L., Puccio, A. M., Poropatic, R., Collins, M. W., & Kontos, A. P. (2014, August). *TEAM TBI: Diagnosis of white matter damage with high definition fiber tracking in patients with chronic TBI.* Paper presented at the Military Health System Research Symposium, Fort Lauderdale, FL.

Schulz, M. R., Marshall, S. W., Mueller, F. O., Yang, J., Weaver, N. L., Kalsbeek, W. D., & Bowling, J. M. (2004). Incidence and risk factors for concussion in high school athletes, North Carolina, 1996–1999. *American Journal of Epidemiology, 160,* 937–944. http://dx.doi.org/10.1093/aje/kwh304

Seidman, D. H., Burlingame, J., Yousif, L. R., Donahue, X. P., Krier, J., Rayes, L. J., . . . Shaw, M. K. (2015). Evaluation of the King-Devick test as a concussion screening tool in high school football players. *Journal of the Neurological Sciences, 356*(1-2), 97–101. http://dx.doi.org/10.1016/j.jns.2015.06.021

Seymour, B. (2013). Defining concussion and mild traumatic brain injury: A history of confusion and debate. *Sound Neuroscience: An Undergraduate Neuroscience Journal, 1*(1), Article 9. Retrieved from http://soundideas.pugetsound.edu/soundneuroscience/vol1/iss1/9

Shapcott, E. J., Bloom, G. A., Johnston, K. M., Loughead, T. M., & Delaney, J. S. (2007). The effects of explanatory style on concussion outcomes in sport. *NeuroRehabilitation, 22,* 161–167.

Sheline, Y. I., Wang, P. W., Gado, M. H., Csernansky, J. G., & Vannier, M. W. (1996). Hippocampal atrophy in recurrent major depression. *Proceedings of the National Academy of Sciences of the United States of America, 93,* 3908–3913. http://dx.doi.org/10.1073/pnas.93.9.3908

Shin, S. S., Pathak, S., Presson, N., Bird, W., Wagener, L., Schneider, W., . . . Fernandez-Miranda, J. C. (2014). Detection of white matter injury in concussion using high-definition fiber tractography. *Progress in Neurological Surgery, 28,* 86–93. http://dx.doi.org/10.1159/000358767

Shumway-Cook, A., & Horak, F. B. (1986). Assessing the influence of sensory interaction of balance. Suggestion from the field. *Physical Therapy, 66,* 1548–1550. http://dx.doi.org/10.1093/ptj/66.10.1548

Shumway-Cook, A., & Woollacott, M. H. (1995). *Motor control: Theory and practical applications.* Baltimore, MD: Lippincott, Williams, & Wilkins.

Silver, J. M. (2012). Effort, exaggeration and malingering after concussion. *Journal of Neurology, Neurosurgery, and Psychiatry, 83*, 836–841. http://dx.doi.org/10.1136/jnnp-2011-302078

Silverberg, N. D., Iverson, G. L., McCrea, M., Apps, J. N., Hammeke, T. A., & Thomas, D. G. (2016). Activity-related symptom exacerbations after pediatric concussion. *JAMA Pediatrics, 170*, 946–953. http://dx.doi.org/10.1001/jamapediatrics.2016.1187

Silverberg, N. D., Luoto, T. M., Öhman, J., & Iverson, G. L. (2014). Assessment of mild traumatic brain injury with the King-Devick Test in an emergency department sample. *Brain Injury, 28*, 1590–1593. http://dx.doi.org/10.3109/02699052.2014.943287

Sim, A., Terryberry-Spohr, L., & Wilson, K. R. (2008). Prolonged recovery of memory functioning after mild traumatic brain injury in adolescent athletes. *Journal of Neurosurgery, 108*, 511–516. http://dx.doi.org/10.3171/JNS/2008/108/3/0511

Slobounov, S., Sebastianelli, W., & Hallett, M. (2012). Residual brain dysfunction observed one year post-mild traumatic brain injury: Combined EEG and balance study. *Clinical Neurophysiology, 123*, 1755–1761. http://dx.doi.org/10.1016/j.clinph.2011.12.022

Snook, M. L., Henry, L. C., Sanfilippo, J. S., Zelznik, A. J., & Kontos, A. P. (2016). A prospective examination of abnormal menstrual patterns in adolescent female athletes following concussion: 3557 June 4, 10:00 AM–10:15 AM. *Medicine and Science in Sports and Exercise, 48*(5, Suppl. 1), 985. http://dx.doi.org/10.1249/01.mss.0000487961.25488.b2

Snook, M. L., Henry, L. C., Sanfilippo, J. S., Zeleznik, A. J., & Kontos, A. P. (2017). Abnormal menstrual patterns in young women following concussion. *JAMA Pediatrics, 171*, 879–886.

Solomon, G. S., Kuhn, A. W., Zuckerman, S. L., Casson, I. R., Viano, D. C., Lovell, M. R., & Sills, A. K. (2016). Participation in pre-high school football and neurological, neuroradiological, and neuropsychological findings in later life: A study of 45 retired national football league players. *The American Journal of Sports Medicine, 44*, 1106–1115. http://dx.doi.org/10.1177/0363546515626164

Solomon, G. S., & Sills, A. (2014). Chronic traumatic encephalopathy and the availability cascade. *The Physician and Sportsmedicine, 42*(3), 26–31. http://dx.doi.org/10.3810/psm.2014.09.2072

Spadoni, A. D., Kosheleva, E., Buchsbaum, M. S., & Simmons, A. N. (2015). Neural correlates of malingering in mild traumatic brain injury: A positron emission tomography study. *Psychiatry Research: Neuroimaging, 233*, 367–372. http://dx.doi.org/10.1016/j.pscychresns.2015.06.007

Stamm, J. M., Bourlas, A. P., Baugh, C. M., Fritts, N. G., Daneshvar, D. H., Martin, B. M., . . . Stern, R. A. (2015). Age of first exposure to football and later-life cognitive impairment in former NFL players. *Neurology, 84*, 1114–1120. http://dx.doi.org/10.1212/WNL.0000000000001358

Stewart, T. C., Gilliland, J., & Fraser, D. D. (2014). An epidemiologic profile of pediatric concussions: Identifying urban and rural differences. *The Journal of Trauma and Acute Care Surgery, 76,* 736–742. http://dx.doi.org/10.1097/TA.0b013e3182aafdf5

Sufrinko, A., Johnson, E., & Henry, L. (2016). The influence of sleep duration and sleep-related symptoms on baseline neurocognitive performance among male and female high school athletes. *Neuropsychology, 30,* 484–491. http://dx.doi.org/10.1037/neu0000250

Sufrinko, A., McAllister-Deitrick, J., Elbin, R. J., Collins, M. W., & Kontos, A. P. (2018). Familial history of migraine is associated with post-traumatic migraine following sport-related concussion in adolescents. *Journal of Head Trauma Rehabilitation, 33,* 7–14.

Sufrinko, A., Pearce, K., Elbin, R. J., Covassin, T., Johnson, E., Collins, M., & Kontos, A. P. (2015). The effect of preinjury sleep difficulties on neurocognitive impairment and symptoms after sport-related concussion. *The American Journal of Sports Medicine, 43,* 830–838. http://dx.doi.org/10.1177/0363546514566193

Sussman, E. S., Ho, A. L., Pendharkar, A. V., & Ghajar, J. (2016). Clinical evaluation of concussion: The evolving role of oculomotor assessments. *Journal of Neurosurgery: Neurosurgical Focus, 40,* E7. http://dx.doi.org/10.3171/2016.1.FOCUS15610

Svensson, M., Lexell, J., & Deierborg, T. (2015). Effects of physical exercise on neuroinflammation, neuroplasticity, neurodegeneration, and behavior: What we can learn from animal models in clinical settings. *Neurorehabilitation and Neural Repair, 29,* 577–589. http://dx.doi.org/10.1177/1545968314562108

Swan, A., Nichols, S., Drake, A., Angeles, A., Diwakar, M., Song, T., . . . Huang, M. X. (2015). Magnetoencephalography slow-wave detection in patients with mild traumatic brain injury and ongoing symptoms correlated with long-term neuropsychological outcome. *Journal of Neurotrauma, 32,* 1510–1521. http://dx.doi.org/10.1089/neu.2014.3654

Tate, C. M., Wang, K. K., Eonta, S., Zhang, Y., Carr, W., Tortella, F. C., . . . Kamimori, G. H. (2013). Serum brain biomarker level, neurocognitive performance, and self-reported symptom changes in soldiers repeatedly exposed to low-level blast: A breacher pilot study. *Journal of Neurotrauma, 30,* 1620–1630. http://dx.doi.org/10.1089/neu.2012.2683

Terrell, T. R., Bostick, R. M., Abramson, R., Xie, D., Barfield, W., Cantu, R., . . . Ewing, T. (2008). APOE, APOE promoter, and Tau genotypes and risk for concussion in college athletes. *Clinical Journal of Sports Medicine, 18,* 10–17.

Theadom, A., Parag, V., Dowell, T., McPherson, K., Starkey, N., Barker-Collo, S., . . . Feigin, V. L., & the BIONIC Research Group. (2016). Persistent problems 1 year after mild traumatic brain injury: A longitudinal population study in New Zealand. *The British Journal of General Practice, 66*(642), e16–e23. http://dx.doi.org/10.3399/bjgp16X683161

Thiagarajan, P., & Ciuffreda, K. J. (2014). Versional eye tracking in mild traumatic brain injury (mTBI): Effects of oculomotor training (OMT). *Brain Injury, 28,* 930–943. http://dx.doi.org/10.3109/02699052.2014.888761

Thiagarajan, P., & Ciuffreda, K. J. (2015). Short-term persistence of oculomotor rehabilitative changes in mild traumatic brain injury (mTBI): A pilot study of clinical effects. *Brain Injury, 29*, 1475–1479. http://dx.doi.org/10.3109/02699052.2015.1070905

Thiagarajan, P., Ciuffreda, K. J., Capo-Aponte, J. E., Ludlam, D. P., & Kapoor, N. (2014). Oculomotor neurorehabilitation for reading in mild traumatic brain injury (mTBI): An integrative approach. *NeuroRehabilitation, 34*(1), 129–146.

Thomas, D. G., Apps, J. N., Hoffmann, R. G., McCrea, M., & Hammeke, T. (2015). Benefits of strict rest after acute concussion: A randomized controlled trial. *Pediatrics, 135*(2), 213–223. http://dx.doi.org/10.1542/peds.2014-0966

Tierney, R. T., Mansell, J. L., Higgins, M., McDevitt, J. K., Toone, N., Gaughan, J. P., . . . Krynetskiy, E. (2010). Apolipoprotein E genotype and concussion in college athletes. *Clinical Journal of Sport Medicine, 20*, 464–468. http://dx.doi.org/10.1097/JSM.0b013e3181fc0a81

Tierney, R. T., Sitler, M. R., Swanik, C. B., Swanik, K. A., Higgins, M., & Torg, J. (2005). Gender differences in head-neck segment dynamic stabilization during head acceleration. *Medicine and Science in Sports and Exercise, 37*(2), 272–279. http://dx.doi.org/10.1249/01.MSS.0000152734.47516.AA

Tkachenko, N., Singh, K., Hasanaj, L., Serrano, L., & Kothare, S. V. (2016). Sleep disorders associated with mild traumatic brain injury using Sport Concussion Assessment Tool 3. *Pediatric Neurology, 57*, 46–50.

Tombaugh, T. N. (1997). The Test of Memory Malingering (TOMM): Normative data from cognitively intact and cognitively impaired individuals. *Psychological Assessment, 9*, 260–268.

Treleaven, J. (2011). Dizziness, unsteadiness, visual disturbances, and postural control: Implications for the transition to chronic symptoms after a whiplash trauma. *Spine, 36*(Suppl. 25), S211–S217. http://dx.doi.org/10.1097/BRS.0b013e3182387f78

Tysvaer, A. T., & Løchen, E. A. (1991). Soccer injuries to the brain. A neuropsychologic study of former soccer players. *The American Journal of Sports Medicine, 19*(1), 56–60. http://dx.doi.org/10.1177/036354659101900109

Tysvaer, A. T., & Storli, O. (1981). Association football injuries to the brain. A preliminary report. *British Journal of Sports Medicine, 15*(3), 163–166. http://dx.doi.org/10.1136/bjsm.15.3.163

UPMC Sports Medicine Concussion Program. (2017). *Rethink concussion*. Retrieved from http://rethinkconcussions.upmc.com/

Valovich McLeod, T. C., & Hale, T. D. (2015). Vestibular and balance issues following sport-related concussion. *Brain Injury, 29*(2), 175–184. http://dx.doi.org/10.3109/02699052.2014.965206

Valovich, T. C., Perrin, D. H., & Gansneder, B. M. (2003). Repeat administration elicits a practice effect with the balance error scoring system but not with the standardized assessment of concussion in high school athletes. *Journal of Athletic Training, 38*(1), 51–56.

Vanhelst, J., Beghin, L., Duhamel, A., Manios, Y., Molnar, D., De Henauw, S., . . . Healthy Lifestyle in Europe by Nutrition in Adolescence Study Group. (2016). Physical activity is associated with attention capacity in adolescents. *Journal of Pediatrics, 168*, 126–131.

Vaughan, C. G., Gerst, E. H., Sady, M. D., Newman, J. B., & Gioia, G. A. (2014). The relation between testing environment and baseline performance in child and adolescent concussion assessment. *American Journal of Sports Medicine, 42*, 1716–1723.

Vedaa, O. W. S., West Saxvig, I., Wilhelmsen-Langeland, A., Bjorvatn, B., & Pallesen, S. (2012). School start time, sleepiness and function in Norwegian adolescents. *Scandinavian Journal of Educational Research, 56*(1), 55–67. http://dx.doi.org/10.1080/00313831.2011.567396

Walker, L. S., Beck, J. E., Garber, J., & Lambert, W. (2009). The Children's Somatization Inventory: Psychometric properties of the revised form (CSI-24). *Journal of Pediatric Psychology, 34*, 430–440.

Walker, L. S., & Garber, J. (2003). *Manual for the Children's Somatization Inventory*. Nashville, TN: Vanderbilt University Medical Center.

Walker, W. C., Franke, L. M., McDonald, S. D., Sima, A. P., & Keyser-Marcus, L. (2015). Prevalence of mental health conditions after military blast exposure, their co-occurrence, and their relation to mild traumatic brain injury. *Brain Injury, 29*(13-14), 1581–1588. http://dx.doi.org/10.3109/02699052.2015.1075151

Wang, K. K., Ottens, A. K., Liu, M. C., Lewis, S. B., Meegan, C., Oli, M. W., . . . Hayes, R. L. (2005). Proteomic identification of biomarkers of traumatic brain injury. *Expert Review of Proteomics, 2*, 603–614. http://dx.doi.org/10.1586/14789450.2.4.603

Wells, E. M., Goodkin, H. P., & Griesbach, G. S. (2016). Challenges in determining the role of rest and exercise in the management of mild traumatic brain injury. *Journal of Child Neurology, 31*(1), 86–92. http://dx.doi.org/10.1177/0883073815570152

Wickwire, E. M., Williams, S. G., Roth, T., Capaldi, V. F., Jaffe, M., Moline, M., . . . Lettieri, C. J. (2016). Sleep, sleep disorders, and mild traumatic brain injury. What we know and what we need to know: Findings from a national working group. *Neurotherapeutics; The Journal of the American Society for Experimental NeuroTherapeutics, 13*, 403–417. http://dx.doi.org/10.1007/s13311-016-0429-3

Wiese-Bjornstal, D., Smith, A., Shaffer, S., & Morrey, M. (1998). An integrated model of response to sport injury: Psychological and sociological dynamics. *Journal of Applied Sport Psychology, 10*(1), 46–49. http://dx.doi.org/10.1080/10413209808406377

Williams, J., & Andersen, M. (1998). Psychosocial antecedents of sport injury: Review and critique of the stress and injury model. *Journal of Applied Sport Psychology, 10*, 5–25. http://dx.doi.org/10.1080/10413209808406375

Williams, R. M., Welch, C. E., Weber, M. L., Parsons, J. T., & Valovich McLeod, T. C. (2014). Athletic trainers' management practices and referral patterns for adolescent athletes after sport-related concussion. *Sports Health, 6,* 434–439. http://dx.doi.org/10.1177/1941738114545612

Withington, E. T. (Trans.). (1928). *Hippocrates: Vol. III. On wounds in the head* (Loeb Classical Library, No. 149). Cambridge, MA: Harvard University Press.

Wojtys, E. M., Hovda, D., Landry, G., Boland, A., Lovell, M., McCrea, M., & Minkoff, J. (1999). Concussion in sports. *The American Journal of Sports Medicine, 27,* 676–687. http://dx.doi.org/10.1177/03635465990270052401

Womble, M. N., McAllister-Deitrick, J., Reynolds, E., Collins, M., Elbin, R., & Kontos, A. (2017). *Role of pre and post-injury risk factors in predicting vestibular-oculomotor outcomes following concussion.* Manuscript under review.

Womble, M. N., Reynolds, E., Schatz, P., Shah, K. M., & Kontos, A. P. (2016). Test–retest reliability of computerized neurocognitive testing in youth ice hockey players. *Archives of Clinical Neuropsychology, 31,* 305–312. http://dx.doi.org/10.1093/arclin/acw011

Wood, R. L., O'Hagan, G., Williams, C., McCabe, M., & Chadwick, N. (2014). Anxiety sensitivity and alexithymia as mediators of postconcussion syndrome following mild traumatic brain injury. *Journal of Head Trauma and Rehabilitation, 29,* E9–E17.

Woodrome, S. E., Yeates, K. O., Taylor, H. G., Rusin, J., Bangert, B., Dietrich, A., . . . Wright, M. (2011). Coping strategies as a predictor of post-concussive symptoms in children with mild traumatic brain injury versus mild orthopedic injury. *Journal of the International Neuropsychological Society, 17,* 317–326. http://dx.doi.org/10.1017/S1355617710001700

Wrisley, D. M., Marchetti, G. F., Kuharsky, D. K., & Whitney, S. L. (2004). Reliability, internal consistency, and validity of data obtained with the functional gait assessment. *Physical Therapy, 84,* 906–918.

Yang, J., Peek-Asa, C., Covassin, T., & Torner, J. C. (2015). Post-concussion symptoms of depression and anxiety in division I collegiate athletes. *Developmental Neuropsychology, 40*(1), 18–23. http://dx.doi.org/10.1080/87565641.2014.973499

Yuh, E. L., Hawryluk, G. W., & Manley, G. T. (2014). Imaging concussion: A review. *Neurosurgery, 75*(Suppl. 4), S50–S63. http://dx.doi.org/10.1227/NEU.0000000000000491

Zemek, R., Barrowman, N., Freedman, S. B., Gravel, J., Gagnon, I., McGahern, C., . . . Osmond, M. H., & the Pediatric Emergency Research Canada Concussion Team. (2016). Clinical risk score for persistent postconcussion symptoms among children with acute concussion in the ED. *Journal of the American Medical Association, 315,* 1014–1025. http://dx.doi.org/10.1001/jama.2016.1203

Zhang, M. R., Red, S. D., Lin, A. H., Patel, S. S., & Sereno, A. B. (2013). Evidence of cognitive dysfunction after soccer playing with ball heading using a novel tablet-based approach. *PLoS One, 8*(2), e57364. http://dx.doi.org/10.1371/journal.pone.0057364

Zhang, Z., Larner, S. F., Kobeissy, F., Hayes, R. L., & Wang, K. K. (2010). Systems biology and theranostic approach to drug discovery and development to treat traumatic brain injury. *Methods in Molecular Biology, 662,* 317–329. http://dx.doi.org/10.1007/978-1-60761-800-3_16

Zuckerbraun, N. S., Atabaki, S., Collins, M. W., Thomas, D., & Gioia, G. A. (2014). Use of modified acute concussion evaluation tools in the emergency department. *Pediatrics, 133,* 635–642. http://dx.doi.org/10.1542/peds.2013-2600

INDEX

ABOUT THE AUTHORS

Anthony P. Kontos, PhD, is the research director for the University of Pittsburgh Medical Center Sports Medicine Concussion Program, where he also directs the Concussion Research Laboratory. He is an associate professor in the Department of Orthopaedic Surgery at the University of Pittsburgh. He received his doctoral degree in kinesiology/sport psychology from Michigan State University, where he also received master's degrees in counseling psychology and exercise science and completed an internship in counseling psychology. He completed his bachelor of arts degree in psychology at Adrian College, where he was a 4-year starter on the men's soccer team. His research focuses on neurocognitive, neuromotor, and psychological effects of concussion in sport, pediatric, and military populations. He has more than 180 professional publications and 270 professional presentations, and he has received research funding from the National Institutes of Health, U.S. Department of Defense, National Collegiate Athletic Association, National Football League/General Electric Head Health Challenge, and U.S. Army Special Operations Command. Dr. Kontos served as chair of the Sub-acute Subgroup on the NIH Sports Concussion Common Data Elements working group, attended the 2014 White House Healthy Kids and Safe Sports

Concussion Summit, and codirected the 2015 Targeted Evaluation and Active Management Approach to Treating Concussion meeting in Pittsburgh. He is also past president and fellow of the American Psychological Association's Division 47 (Society for Sport, Exercise and Performance Psychology).

Michael (Micky) W. Collins, PhD, is executive and clinical director for the University of Pittsburgh Medical Center Sports Medicine Concussion Program and an associate professor of orthopaedic surgery at the University of Pittsburgh. He directs six clinical sites with more than 18,000 patient visits annually for concussion and related issues. A graduate of the University of Southern Maine with a bachelor's degree in psychology and biology in 1991, Dr. Collins earned a master's degree in psychology in 1995 and a doctoral degree in clinical psychology in 1998 at Michigan State University. He has specialized in concussion research for the past 17 years; he has published more than 90 peer-reviewed articles and delivered more than 350 presentations at national and international meetings. He has received funding from the Centers for Disease Control and Prevention, U.S. Department of Defense, National Institutes of Health, National Football League/General Electric, and the U.S. Army Special Operations Command. Dr. Collins has been the recipient of several honors, including the Innovations in Treatment Award from the North American Brain Injury Society, the 2010 National Council on Brain Injury annual award for outstanding research and advocacy, and the 2007 Annual Butters Award from the National Academy of Neuropsychology. He attended the 2014 White House Healthy Kids and Safe Sports Concussion Summit and chaired the 2015 Targeted Evaluation and Active Management Approach to Treating Concussion meeting in Pittsburgh. An athlete himself, Dr. Collins played in the 1989 National Collegiate Athletic Association Baseball College World Series.